THE GREAT PHYSICIAN'S

R^x *for*

COLDS AND FLU

JORDAN RUBIN

with Joseph Brasco, MD

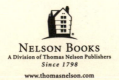

NELSON BOOKS
A Division of Thomas Nelson Publishers
Since 1798

www.thomasnelson.com

Published in Nashville, Tennessee, by Thomas Nelson, Inc.

Nelson Books titles may be purchased in bulk for educational, business, fund-raising, or sales promotional use. For information, please e-mail SpecialMarkets@ThomasNelson.com.

Unless otherwise noted, Scripture quotations are taken from the NEW KING JAMES VERSION®. Copyright © 1979, 1980, 1982 by Thomas Nelson, Inc. Used by permission. All rights reserved.

Library of Congress Cataloging-in-Publication Data

Rubin, Jordan.
    The great physician's Rx for colds and flu / by Jordan Rubin with Joseph Brasco.
      p. cm.
    ISBN 0-7852-1402-X (hardcover)
    1. Cold (Disease)—Prevention—Popular works. 2. Influenza—Prevention—Popular works.
3. Cold (Disease)—Religious aspects—Christianity. 4. Influenza—Religious aspects—
Christianity. I. Brasco, Joseph. II. Title.
RF361.R83 2006
616.2'05—dc22   2006013764

Printed in the United States of America

1 2 3 4 5 QW 10 09 08 07 06

CONTENTS

Introduction: It's Going Around!   v

Key #1: Eat to Live   1

Key #2: Supplement Your Diet with Whole Food   23
      Nutritionals, Living Nutrients, and Superfoods

Key #3: Practice Advanced Hygiene   40

Key #4: Condition Your Body with Exercise   50
      and Body Therapies

Key #5: Reduce Toxins in Your Environment   57

Key #6: Avoid Deadly Emotions   65

Key #7: Live a Life of Prayer and Purpose   69

The Great Physician's Rx for Colds and Flu Battle Plan   75

Notes   95

About the Authors   99

INTRODUCTION

It's Going Around!

Bird flu, anyone?

I know that attention spans are short-lived these days, but you had to have been sleeping against a tree trunk like Rip Van Winkle not to catch the media's full-court press last winter. "Experts Fear Bird Flu But Can't Predict Timing," proclaimed a Knight Ridder News Service headline. "Race to Prevent Global Epidemic," declared *Newsweek* while picturing a sick-looking, beady-headed red rooster on the cover. Not since Alfred Hitchcock released *The Birds*, a frightening film from the early '60s, have our fine feathered friends been held in such ill repute.

What the mainstream media was doing was working from a template, and with bird flu, the stories generally followed this outline:

1. Something bad is happening in Asia, and it could spread to our borders.

2. Experts are concerned that one of the worst natural disasters in the history of mankind could . . . just might . . . happen very soon.

3. The U.S. government doesn't want to be caught short, so measures are being taken to protect the public health.

4. Despite anyone's well-intentioned efforts, we're doomed, unless science can develop a vaccine.

These feature articles were often accompanied by a grainy sepia-toned World War I–era photo of a cavernous, wood-raftered emergency hospital in Camp Funston, Kansas, where hundreds of bed-ridden victims lay on rows of cots while being nursed back to health. A cutline would state that an estimated 670,000 Americans died from the "Spanish flu" influenza pandemic of 1918–1919.

I harbor no doubts that 1918 was not a good time to catch the flu. The influenza pandemic of 1918–1919 killed many more U.S. soldiers than the gruesome trench warfare of World War I. Historians are divided on how many perished globally from the massive influenza outbreak, but estimates run between 20 million and 50 million. In the U.S., one-fourth of the population was infected; globally, 20 percent were tainted with the influenza. My good friend and writer, Mike Yorkey, lost his great-grandfather to the 1918 influenza outbreak.

The Allies of World War I dubbed the epidemic the "Spanish Flu," probably because the outbreak received greater press attention in Spain since the Spanish stood on the sidelines during World War I and enacted no wartime censorship. When Spain was hit hard by an early outbreak of the disease, other countries were eager to pin the epidemic tail on its behind, although some thought the Germans—who introduced poisonous mustard gas on the Western Front in 1915—were behind a diabolical plot to exterminate their enemies with another form of biological warfare.

The Spanish flu quickly traversed the Atlantic and reached our shores, thanks to the human cargo aboard troop transport ships and trading vessels. Like an invading force, it didn't take long for the Spanish Flu to establish a beachhead in our major cities. As body counts rose and state and local authorities realized they had a modern-day plague on their hands, severe restrictions were placed on public gatherings and travel. Theaters, dance halls, churches, and other public gathering places were shut down. Quarantines were enforced. Funerals were limited to fifteen minutes.

Many of these public restrictions were entirely appropriate measures. Once "La Grippe"—the other name associated with the 1918 flu—clutched you by your sore throat, you could be a goner, especially if you were between the ages of twenty and forty. For some reason, the Grim Reaper wielded its sickle on those in the prime of their lives, not young children or the elderly. Victim's lungs filled rapidly, and they struggled to clear their airways of a blood-tinged froth that gushed from their noses and mouths. What happened is that you essentially drowned yourself in a matter of days or even hours.

Ghastly. Physicians were helpless against an epidemic that historians today call the most devastating ever—causing far more deaths than the Black Death Bubonic Plague from 1347 to 1351, although it must be noted that many more people were living at the turn of the twentieth century than 650 years ago.[1] Since the Spanish flu was an indiscriminate affliction that cut across economic and social lines, fatalism ruled the day, which was encapsulated in a rhyme that children sang as they skipped rope in 1918:

I had a little bird
Its name was Enza
I opened the window
And in-flu-enza

The suspected source of the 1918–1919 flu pandemic was a bird flu that jumped directly to humans, morphed into a human virus, and then was spread from one person to another. Could that happen again today? No one is sure, which is why we're seeing so much media speculation. *60 Minutes* correspondent Steve Kroft said, "The World Health Organization calls [the bird flu] the most serious health threat facing the planet, greater than AIDS or tuberculosis." Kroft made this statement because public-health authorities are gravely concerned that a deadly bird flu virus could make that critical leap to human-to-human transmission.[2]

As Hall of Fame catcher Yogi Berra once said, if that happens, it would be déjà vu all over again.

NOTHING TO SNEEZE AT

So is another deadly bird flu pandemic on the horizon?

I'm not qualified to answer that, but many leading health experts have been saying that it's not a question of if, but when. Their concerns are based on the recent discovery of a lethal virus named H5N1, which was responsible for the death of 140 million birds in Asia recently, a number that includes those intentionally killed to stop the spread of the virus. Since 2003, a

couple hundred unfortunate souls have contracted H5N1—
mainly because they were in close contact with either the drop-
pings or blood of domestic poultry. *Half* of those infected have
died, which has lit a fire under public-health authorities to
sound the alarm. In the fall of 2005, researchers genetically
linked H5N1 to the 1918 influenza pandemic.

Hence the official concern, although if H5N1 mutated into
a human virus, it would turn less deadly. "That's because it
would have to mutate or combine with another virus, which
would almost certainly lower its killing efficiency," wrote Emily
Flynn Vencat in *Newsweek* magazine. "The terrifying 1918 bug,
for example, killed only one in one hundred . . . but 'no virus
under the sun would be able to spread with that kind of mortality,' says John Oxford a virologist at Queen Mary's School of
Medicine in London."[3]

Now everyone is watching to see if the bird virus—also
known as avian flu—can be passed from person to person. So far,
that hasn't happened, which is why we dodged a germ-covered
bullet during the winter of 2005–2006. If the nasty bird flu gets
rolling in the future, however, epidemiologists predict that the
death toll could be 2.5 percent of the world's population, or 150
million people. An intercontinental spread of bird flu would
leap across borders like an out-of-control brush fire, invoking
international havoc and wrecking the global economy.

I think we need to be concerned, even though the media has
cried wolf many times over the years about the next "epidemic"
that could kill millions. Since colds and flu are the most common form of illness, it behooves us to remain vigilant and take

steps to protect ourselves. We should be encouraged by the fact that avian flu has been circulating in China for more than a dozen years without jumping into human population.

This book, *The Great Physician's Rx for Colds and Flu*, however, is about much more than H5N1 and whether our public-health authorities can protect us. I'm confident that the chances of catching a *life-threatening* flu, cold, or sinus condition are remote, for which I thank the Lord. What I want to address are the *regular* colds and everyday flu bugs that knock us off our feet, make us feel awful, and stop us from being productive at home, in ministry, and at work.

Colds and flu are viral illnesses that share many of the same symptoms and are caused by the same family of respiratory viruses, although there are some key differences. A cold is an infection of the upper respiratory tract that includes a runny nose, sneezing, and coughing. The flu usually features the same symptoms, only more severe, along with fever, muscle aches, and more persistent coughing.[4] Flu sufferers will sometimes experience spikes of high fever followed by chills, which can exhaust victims and cause their whole body to feel sore. Here's my amateur, nonmedical description of the differences between a cold and the flu: When you have a cold, you can still go to work, do your chores, or carry on with a normal day. When you have the flu, you're down for the count and too weak to get out of bed.

According to the Mayo Clinic, the average American adult contracts between two and four upper respiratory illnesses a year—mostly during the "cold and flu season" between October and April. School-aged children, as any parent knows, are more susceptible since they're cooped up with twenty or thirty class-mates every day; they average between six and ten colds a year.[5]

The economic and societal impact of colds and flu is nothing to sneeze at. The most frequent illness among Americans, these viral illnesses annually attack 500 million times and cost $40 billion in doctor's bills, medication, and missed work and school days, a University of Michigan study reports.[6] According to the National Institute of Allergy and Infectious Diseases (NIAID), some estimates put the number of colds as high as $1 billion a year.[7] Catching a flu bug is less common but poses a more serious health threat: as many as 36,000 Americans die each year from complications relating to the flu, and more than 200,000 experience such respiratory difficulties that they must be hospitalized.[8]

The so-called common cold is aptly named because in a given year, nearly half of the United States' population will catch a cold, and 40 percent will develop influenza.[9] The waiting rooms of family physicians are filled during the height of the cold-and-flu season with young and old and everyone in between sneezing, sniffling, and blowing their noses.

Chilly weather has nothing to do with whether you get a cold. Researchers believe that the back-to-school influx in the fall provides a fine laboratory for the exchange of viruses. The climate change to colder weather also causes people to stay indoors, which increases their chances of being in close, physical proximity to a family member or friend with a viral condition. When people sneeze, wipe their runny nose on their fingers, or cough, they put you in a position to catch a cold from one of two hundred or so rhinoviruses that take up residence in your nose, or "rhino" in medicalese. After parking themselves in your nasal cavity, these rhinoviruses go to work infecting the rest of your body as they replicate themselves by the billions. Before you know it, you're sniffling and sneezing, and unless your body's immune system can repel these invaders, you're battling a cold.

Upon infection, your body becomes a virus-making factory for a day or two as the guest virus replicates itself over and over and over. Once a cold has you in its grip, it's difficult to throw it off in less than two days. Most of the time, the aches, the sore throat, the runny nose, the scratchy throat, and the hacking cough usually hang around for three to ten days, and residual coughing can last another two or three weeks. Flu viruses tend to be stronger than those of colds, but both are highly contagious and passed along by a sneeze, cough, or kiss.

CONVENTIONAL TREATMENT

Once the virus establishes a beachhead in your respiratory tract, you'll know it because you feel lousy right away. When you feel lousy, you usually do something about it, but initial treatment depends on how you were raised.

You may run for the medicine cabinet like Mom did, where an array of half-used bottles of syrups, lozenges, sprays, and pills from your *last* cold have gathered dust. This colorful collection of aspirins, nasal decongestants, cough suppressants, and antihistamines are among the dozens of cold and flu remedies sold over the counter at pharmacies and supermarkets. Heavily advertised, relatively inexpensive, and endorsed by lab-coated health professionals on TV and in print ads, these over-the-counter drugs (OTCs) contain analgesics such as acetaminophen, aspirin, and ibuprofen, antihistamines, and nasal decongestants. Analgesics relieve aches and pains and reduce fever. Antihistamines dry up a runny nose, but these products may make you drowsy. (I know some people who use Benadryl, a popular antihistamine, to help them get over jet lag.) Nasal decongestants unstuff nasal passages.

A University of Michigan study found that Americans spend $2.9 billion on over-the-counter cold medications, $400 million on prescription drugs, and more than $1 billion on antibiotics, which should only be taken if a bacterial complication develops.[10] The efficacy of OTC drugs is a subject of research and debate in the scientific community. No one is pretending that a couple of Excedrin PMs or a one-ounce cup of cherry-flavored NyQuil will shoo away a cold or knock down a flu right away, but many feel these medicaments shorten the duration of the illness.

When stronger cold- or flu-like symptoms—vomiting, high fever, shaking chills, painful swallowing, persistent coughing, and coughing up thick, yellow-green mucus—fail to diminish, plan B is seeing the doctor. Besides reminding you to drink plenty of liquids and get plenty of rest, family physicians don't have a lot of weapons against colds and the flu in their arsenal besides writing you a prescription that attacks the virus and stops it from spreading to the rest of your family. The most popular prescription these days is for Tamiflu (oseltamivir), but

Flumadine (rimantadine) and Symmetrel (amantadine) can also be prescribed, although the latter two are known for producing unpleasant side effects such as light-headedness and inability to sleep. These antiviral medicines must be taken within forty-eight hours of the onset of flu symptoms to be effective.

Many Americans don't wait for the flu to hit before doing something. Each fall and early winter, more than sixty-five million line up at workplaces, warehouse clubs, drugstores, and local clinics, roll up a sleeve, and endure a pinprick to receive their annual flu shot. The flu shot is a vaccine containing influenza viruses grown in chicken eggs each year. Scientists make a different vaccine each year because the strains of flu viruses change rapidly, and the U.S. Centers for Disease Control (CDC) recommends that people sixty-five years and older, those in nursing homes, pregnant women, children between six and twenty-three months old, and those with compromised immune systems get a flu shot each fall. The CDC believes that the flu vaccine prevents influenza in about 70–90 percent of healthy persons younger than sixty-five years of age, but points out that an unpredicted new viral strain may appear after the vaccine has been made, meaning all bets are off the table. The FDA has recently approved a nasal spray flu vaccine called FluMist, which is available in doctor's offices. FluMist is not recommended for those with lung conditions, diabetes, kidney dysfunction, or for those who are pregnant.

I have chosen never to get a flu shot, or the new FluMist, because I don't personally believe in artificially stimulating the immune system in order to avoid the flu. I would never try to talk anyone out of having an annual flu shot; that's a personal decision that must be carefully weighed. Every vaccine comes with side effects, sometimes large, sometimes small. As mentioned, getting the flu shot each fall doesn't guarantee immunity over the winter months since there are many flu strains that are constantly mutating. There are pros and cons to flu shots, but as for myself, I prefer to keep my immune system healthy in other ways.

ALTERNATIVE TREATMENTS

If there was ever a health condition that had the most home remedies, it would definitely be colds and flu. Some of the ones I've heard about include gargling salt water, drinking grapefruit juice by the quart, submitting to acupuncture, and employing horsetail (the herb) inhalations.

Maybe some of them work. I was rarely sick growing up, but on the few occasions when I caught a cold, Mom served up a heaping helping of "Jewish penicillin," otherwise known as homemade chicken soup. (I was raised in a Messianic Jewish home, but with a last name of Rubin, I'm sure you figured that out.) There's something about slurping a zesty soup made from scratch with fiber-rich vegetables such as celery, carrots, onion, and zucchini. I'll have more to say about homemade chicken soup in the next chapter.

Herbs have a long history of being beneficial for treating colds and flu since they stimulate the immune system and have antiviral properties. Some of the herbs commonly used to fight colds and flu are zinc, echinacea, goldenseal, licorice, elderberry, shitake extract, and astragalus. The herb with the greatest amount of scientific support is echinacea, which comes in different delivery systems.

The Encyclopedia of Natural Medicine points out that there have been over three hundred scientific investigations on the immune-enhancing effects of echinacea, including one showing that those taking a 900-milligram dose each day showed a significant reduction of cold symptoms compared to those who took a placebo.[11] *Prescription for Nutritional Healing* points out that zinc lozenges and goldenseal boost the immune system, cat's claw eases cold symptoms, elderberry promotes sweating that can break a fever, and ginger, pau d'arco (a bark from a Brazilian tree), slippery elm, and yarrow tea make you feel better.[12]

Many in alternative medicine suggest taking vitamin C in mega-amounts—2,000 to 20,000 milligrams a day versus the recommended daily values of just 60 milligrams a day—as a way to reduce the incidence, severity, and duration of colds and flu. I'll have more to say about vitamin C therapy in Key #2, but ascorbic acid, an isolated component molecularly similar to the active compound in vitamin C, is said to increase interferon, which is a group of proteins released by white blood cells to combat a virus.

A ROAD MAP FROM HERE

Colds and flu have a nasty way of defying cure or prevention, but I'm confident that following the Great Physician's prescription for colds and flu can speed recovery and minimize the general malaise, coughs, fever, headache, and upper respiratory tract and nasal congestion. I'm not going to sit here and tell you that I've gone ten years without getting a cold, and the flu hasn't laid a glove on me in years. I get sick just like you because I cannot avoid them.

I blame my respiratory illnesses on two things: all the traveling I must do and all the hands I must shake. I take a plane trip at least once a week, and breathing all that recirculated air has to be like walking into an influenza ward at the hospital. Since I speak often and do book signings, I also meet and greet hundreds of people each week. On top of those things, I know that I don't get enough rest. I have a two-year-old son who wakes me up early at home, and when I'm on the road, I have a jam-packed schedule that starts with breakfast meetings and ends with my giving a health seminar or speaking at an evening church service. What I can tell you is that I minimize the incidences of colds and flu and usually miss no more than a day of work per year.

I believe a cold or flu is not something you catch. When your body builds up enough toxic material and reaches a certain threshold, the symptoms of a cold or flu are the body's way of eliminating the breeding ground where these germs live. Mucus is that breeding ground, so when you have the urge to sneeze or blow your nose, your body is discharging mucus and eliminating the germs it collected en masse. I think the best thing is to let it flow because you're getting rid of the junk that's built up in your body. Just keep a box of tissues handy and keep blowing that nose!

People think the cold-and-flu season is the time when you catch a cold and have all these symptoms, but in reality, it's the other way around: you've accumulated enough germs and toxins in the respiratory tract, so the body seeks a way to detoxify, and that's through a sore throat, nasal drip, sneezing, etc. When people get a cold or flu, their first response is to suppress the symptoms; that's why people keep their medicine cabinets filled with over-the-counter medications.

I don't keep any cold medications in the house, and I can't remember the last time I used one. I recommend—and take myself—apple cider vinegar diluted in water and mixed with honey because of its antimicrobial properties. Raw apple cider vinegar, the product of fermented apple juice, is a wonderful combination of tartness and germ-killing acids. When mixed with pure honey and a few ounces of water, the drink becomes a bacteria-killing beverage. I also use a combination of herbs and spices as well as consuming essential oils and CO_2 extracts of herbs and spices with antimicrobial properties. Raw apple cider vinegar is part of the Great Physician's Rx for Colds and Flu Battle Plan (see page 75).

During and after a cold or flu, and every day in between, I consume omega-3 cod-liver oil to make sure I manage inflammation. I also ingest ample amounts of vitamins A and D, which are important for a healthy immune system.

Using the knowledge I've gained on health and nutrition over the years, I can usually cut the duration of my colds and illnesses by days. To use a meteorological metaphor since I live in South Florida—a.k.a. "Hurricane Alley"—when the eye of a cold or flu storm hits my landfall, instead of knocked down by a Category 4 or Category 5 tempest, I get by with a Category 1.

A cure for the common cold hasn't happened for millennia, and I believe it's one of those health conditions that will always be out of reach, even for the most brilliant minds in science. I don't think that means we can't do anything, though. My approach to battling colds and flu is based on 7 Keys to unlock the body's healthy potential that were established in my foundational book *The Great Physician's Rx for Health and Wellness*. These keys are:

Key #1: Eat to Live

Key #2: Supplement Your Diet with Whole Food Nutritionals, Living Nutrients, and Superfoods

Key #3: Practice Advanced Hygiene

Key #4: Condition Your Body with Exercise and Body Therapies

Key #5: Reduce Toxins in Your Environment

Key #6: Avoid Deadly Emotions

Key #7: Live a Life of Prayer and Purpose

Each of these keys should directly support your desire to minimize the effects of wintertime colds and seasonal flu in your life. I know that at the first sign of a sniffle or cough, I practice advanced hygiene right away, drink more water, and *really* pay attention to what I eat.

My main goal for writing *The Great Physician's Rx for Colds and Flu* is to give you a "prevent defense," to use a football term. My seven keys will help you strengthen your immune system and give your body the fuel it needs to beat back viral invaders. Incorporating these timeless principles will allow the living God to transform your health as you honor Him physically, mentally, emotionally, and spiritually.

KEY #1

Eat to Live

Feed a cold, starve a fever."

The proverb is probably as old as Solomon, but some historians believe the adage stems from what a dictionary maker named Withals wrote in 1574: "Fasting is a great remedie of feurer."[1]

Verie interesting. I've read scientific evidence that fasting allows the body to heal and eating eases cold symptoms. A Dutch study performed at the Academic Medical Centre in Amsterdam several years ago attempted to investigate what they called an "old wives' tale," and what they found was that eating and fasting caused brief fluctuations in the amount of two chemical messengers called cytokines. Those who ate stimulated the body's defenses against infection by triggering the releaser of killer white blood cells, which destroy infected cells. Those who fasted had higher concentrations of another cytokine associated with the production of antibodies—the front line of defense against acute infections.[2]

What About Fasting?

Starve a fever?

Sure. I'm a firm believer in the value of giving the body time off while your immune system does battle with the host of viral invaders. My friend Don Colbert, MD,

1

explains in his book, *Fasting Made Easy* (Siloam Press, 2004), that cold and flu symptoms are worsened when we eat while we're sick. Fasting and drinking plenty of water and fresh juices will help your body expel toxic materials through the mucus it creates.

When you're not sick, I think fasting is a superb discipline to incorporate into a healthy lifestyle *and* keep colds and flu at arm's length. When I talk about fasting, I think it's better—and more realistic—to concentrate on completing a one-day partial fast once a week, something I do regularly. For instance, I won't eat breakfast and lunch, so that when I break my fast and eat dinner that night, my body has gone between eighteen and twenty hours without food or sustenance since I last ate dinner the night before. If you've never voluntarily fasted for a day, I urge you to try it—preferably toward the end of the week. I've found that Thursdays or Fridays work best for me because the week is winding down and the weekend is coming up. The benefits are immediate: you'll feel great, get rid of toxins, lose weight, look younger, save money, save time, and become closer to the Lord.

I think the best approach to colds and flu is to follow your gut and listen to your body. If you feel lousy and have no interest in food, then don't eat. If you feel up to a meal, by all means nibble on something . . . healthy, of course.

In this chapter, I'm going to share what I call the "Top Healing Foods" for colds and flu. But for now, I think it would be instructive to talk about what you should eat when you *don't* have a cold or the flu, because what you consume every day impacts your immune system, and *prevention* is the best medicine for a cold or flu. When you keep your immune system healthy, you reduce your susceptibility to catching a cold or flu the next time germs and viruses lodge inside your respiratory system. "People who suffer from more than two colds a year and whose colds last longer than four or five days probably have a weakened immune system," said Michael T. Murray, N.D. "The immune system can be boosted through proper diet, lifestyle, and supplement strategies, and this will help prevent colds from forming in the first place."[3]

"Eating to live," the first key to unlocking your health potential, will enhance your immune system when you follow these two foundational principles:

1. Eat what God created for food.
2. Eat food in a form that is healthy for the body.

Since sneezing, fevers, and coughing usually signify a problem with the immune system, eating foods that God created and were grown, raised, produced, and prepared healthfully is a strong prescription for reducing the ability of one of those two hundred rhinoviruses to successfully attack your body. Eating foods that God created in a form that is healthy for the body means choosing foods as close to the natural source as possible, which will nourish your body, help you perform at optimal levels, and give you the healthiest life possible. Paying attention to the food you eat will help you avoid creating the nutrient deficiencies that lead to illness.

I believe that optimizing nutrition begins with an awareness of what you are sending to your digestive tract. To begin with, everything you put into your mouth is a protein, fat, or carbohydrate. Following correct dietary principles will be key, because each of these nutrients positively or negatively affects your body's cells, which are the front lines of any battle against viral illnesses.

Let's take a closer look at these macronutrients.

THE FIRST WORD ON PROTEINS

Protein, one of the basic components of foods, makes up the essential building blocks of the body, and they are involved in the function of every living cell. One of protein's main tasks is to provide specific nutrient material to grow and repair cells—especially those decimated by a nasty virus.

All proteins are combinations of twenty-two amino acids, which build body organs, muscles, and nerves, to name a few important duties. Your body, however, cannot produce all twenty-two amino acids that you need to live a robust life. Scientists have discovered that eight essential amino acids are missing, meaning that they must come from other sources outside the body. I know the following fact drives vegetarians and vegans crazy, but animal protein—chicken, beef, lamb, fish, dairy, eggs, and so on—is the *only* complete protein source providing the Big Eight amino acids in the right proportions.

I don't believe that the best and most healthy sources of animal protein come from your supermarket's meat case. Commercially raised livestock, fish, and poultry are routinely injected with hormones and fed grain and meal laced with antibiotics, nitrates, and pesticides—chemicals that have been investigated as possible carcinogenic substances. These additives help livestock owners fatten up their herd, which fattens their bottom lines, but these practices may pose health risks to humans who dine on this meat.

The best approach is to eat the healthiest sources of animal protein available, which come from organically raised cattle, sheep, goats, buffalo, and deer—animals that graze on pastureland grasses. Grass-fed meat is leaner and lower in calories than grain-fed meat.

I'm also a huge fan of free-range chicken and eating wild fish captured from lakes, streambeds, or ocean depths. Fish with scales and fins caught in the wild are lean sources of protein and provide all the essential amino acids. Wild fish, which is nutritionally far superior to farm-raised, should be consumed liberally.

ROUNDTABLE ON FATS

God, in His infinite wisdom, created fats as a concentrated source of energy and foundational material for cell membranes and various hormones. Most importantly, healthy fats enhance the immune system but also have a protective effect against heart disease, play a vital role in the health of our bones, protect the liver from alcohol and other toxins, and guard against harmful microorganisms in the digestive tract. Fats add taste to food and provide satiety; otherwise, we would be raiding the refrigerator within an hour of eating if fats didn't give us that full feeling.

The problem with the standard American diet is that people eat too many of the wrong foods containing the wrong fats and not enough of the right foods with the right fats. "Wrong fats" include hydrogenated oils containing trans fats, which raise LDL cholesterol rates, clog arteries, cause heart attacks, and also increase the incidence of most cancers.

As for the "right fats," I'm referring to foods loaded with omega-3 polyunsaturated fats, monounsaturated (omega-9) fatty acids, and conjugated linoleic acid (CLA), as well as healthy saturated fats containing short- and medium-chain fatty acids, such as butter and coconut oil. These good fats are found in a wide range of foods, including salmon, lamb, and goat meat, in dairy products derived from goat's milk, sheep's milk, and cow's milk from organically raised animals, and in flaxseeds, walnuts, olives, macadamia nuts, and avocados. Eating too many of the wrong fats—which are usually found in highly processed foods containing hydrogenated or partially hydrogenated oils—is extremely unhealthy for the body.

My advice is to stay away from packaged dessert treats and store aisles stuffed with processed foods and eat as many foods in their natural state as possible. Eat a couple of organic eggs in the morning. Fill your lunch plate with organic lettuce, tomatoes, and carrots. Snack on raw fruit between meals. At dinner-time, eat a balanced meal of organically produced beef, a more exotic grain like quinoa, and in-season vegetables. When cooking, use butter or extra virgin coconut oil. All of the aforementioned foods are loaded with vitamins, antioxidants, fiber, omega-3 fatty acids, and many micronutrients.

The Truth About Carbohydrates

By definition, carbohydrates are the starches and sugars produced by plant foods, and they are carried in the blood as glucose and regulated by insulin, a hormone that holds the key to the body cell's nutritional door. Thanks to the low-carb diet popularized by Dr. Robert Atkins, Americans have been on a carbohydrate witch hunt for the last five years. The premise behind these trendy books is that burning excess carbohydrates at the stake, so to speak, is the panacea for weight loss.

It's true that reducing the intake of carbohydrates (bread, pasta, rice, pastries, cookies, and cereals, especially those made with processed flours) causes the body to burn excess body fat for fuel and lowers blood sugar and insulin levels. But it's difficult *not* to eat carbs in this country when you look at the standard American diet, which is weighted quite heavily on the carbohydrate side, thanks to the presence of sugar in so many of our processed foods.

Most people eat sugar with every meal: breakfast cereals are frosted with sugar, break time is soda or coffee mixed with sugar and a Danish, lunch has its cookies and treats, and dinner could be sweet-and-sour ribs, sweet potatoes, and corn on the cob, topped off with a sugary dessert. Talk about adding a sweet exclamation point to the day!

A high-sugar diet has always been unhealthy, but research by Nancy Appleton, Ph.D., listed seventy-six ways that sugar can ruin you even if you're in the peak of health. Her first way caught my eye: Dr. Appleton said that sugar suppresses your immune system and impairs your defenses against infectious disease.[4] A high level of sugar in the bloodstream also creates a breeding ground for bacterial growth.

I'm not talking about eliminating all sugar from your diet, because doing so would also mean doing away with God-given foods that contain natural sugars—fruits, vegetables, yogurt, and honey. But severely limiting or entirely avoiding *refined* sugar, which is found in just about every processed food known to man, from store-bought cookies to ketchup, from peanut butter to raspberry jam, from bread to pasta, from colas to sweet teas, is a definite plus for your immune system.

Since most Americans eat foods with refined white flour for every meal, however, be aware that any excess refined carbohydrates, which turn to sugars in the bloodstream, feed normal cells as well as those dangerous viral cells. The key is to boost your immune system by not giving the bad guys the nutrients necessary for growth. Instead, look for carbohydrate foods that are *unrefined*, and the best sources include fruits, vegetables, nuts, seeds, yogurt, honey and grains such as whole wheat, spelt, kamut, quinoa, millet, rye, brown rice, and barley. It's also better to buy organic flour with the words *stone ground, yeast free,* or *sprouted whole grain* on the package label.

Top Healing Foods

We have discussed some healthy foods in this chapter so far, but including the following foods in your diet is a must:

1. Chicken soup. I've had a soft spot in my heart for chicken soup since Mom nursed me back to health with steaming bowls of this hearty meal. The recuperative effects of chicken soup date as far back as the twelfth century when the Jewish physician and philosopher Moses Maimonides recommended its use for the treatment of respiratory infections. These days in Escondido, California, local doctors send patients to Lourdes Mexican Food restaurant to slurp its home-style chicken soup made with "secret spices," and on rainy days, the restaurant sells four hundred bowls of its nourishing soup.[5]

Why is chicken soup so good for the soul? (Hey, that would make a great title to a series of books.) Stephen Rennard, MD, and chief of pulmonary medicine at the University of Nebraska Medical Center in Omaha, says that chicken soup acts as an anti-inflammatory, meaning that sipping chicken soup reduces the inflammation that occurs when coughs and congestion strike the respiratory tract. In addition, chicken soup keeps a check on inflammatory white blood cells, also known as neutrophils, that are produced by the onset of cold symptoms.

Dr. Rennard conducted a full-blown study on the medicinal qualities of chicken soup. He had his wife prepare up a batch using a recipe from her Lithuanian grandmother. Then he carted the homemade chicken soup to his laboratory, where he combined some of the soup with neutrophils to see what would happen. Remember that neutrophils, or white blood cells, rush to attack an invading virus, and that is what causes fluids to build up in the chest.

As Dr. Rennard suspected, his wife's homemade chicken soup demonstrated that neutrophils showed less of a tendency to congregate, but at the same time, these neutrophils did not lose any of their ability to fight off germs.[6] His findings were published in the peer-reviewed journal of the American College of Chest Physicians.[7]

Dr. Rennard also tested more than a dozen store-bought soups, and a third of them slowed down neutrophils even *more*. I'm mystified how that happened since I think you can do better than rushing to the supermarket and purchasing a couple of cans of iconic Campbell's Chicken Noodle Soup. You'll be better off making the real deal from scratch, and you may want to even consider adding chicken feet to the recipe, which Jewish folklore considers the secret to a successful broth. As you look over the following recipe for chicken soup, take notice of the last ingredient I added to this recipe—cayenne pepper. That'll clear the sinuses!

Here's an excellent recipe for chicken soup, which was inspired by my grandma Rose and good friend Sally Fallon, author of *Nourishing Traditions:*

COLD AND FLU BUSTIN' SPICY CHICKEN SOUP

Ingredients:
1 whole chicken (free range, pastured, or organic)
2–4 chicken feet (optional)
3–4 quarts cold filtered water

1 tablespoon raw apple cider vinegar
4 medium-sized onions, coarsely chopped
8 carrots, peeled and coarsely chopped
6 celery stalks, coarsely chopped
2–4 zucchinis, chopped
4–6 tablespoons extra virgin coconut oil
1 bunch parsley
5 garlic cloves
4 inches grated ginger
2–4 tablespoons Celtic Sea Salt
1/4–1/2 teaspoon cayenne pepper

Directions: If you are using a whole chicken, remove fat glands and the gizzards from the cavity. By all means, use chicken feet if you can find them. Place chicken or chicken pieces in a large stainless steel pot with the water, vinegar, and all vegetables except parsley. Let stand for ten minutes before heating. Bring to a boil and remove scum that rises to the top. Cover and cook for twelve to twenty-four hours. The longer you cook the stock, the more healing it will be. About fifteen minutes before finishing the stock, add parsley. This will impart additional mineral ions to the broth.

Remove from heat and take out the chicken and the chicken feet. Let it cool and remove chicken meat from the carcass, discarding the bones and the feet. Drop the meat back in the soup.

2. Coconut milk and coconut oil. You may be scratching your head and saying, "Huh?" Stop scratching. Coconut milk and oil are rich in lauric acid, which is known for being antiviral, antibacterial, and antifungal. The body converts the lauric acid into monolaurin, which is a potent antiviral. Coconut oil also contains capric and caprylic acid, which are medium-chain fatty acids that are antifungal. Even though the flu is not a fungus, killing excess fungi in the body will help improve the immune system, making the body less susceptible to colds and flu.

Don't believe any negative press about coconut oil because of its high level of saturated fat. Modern research is showing that not all saturated fats are the same, and the medium-chain fatty acids do not raise serum cholesterol or contribute to heart disease. I urge you to cook and bake with extra virgin coconut oil, which is a miracle food that few people have ever heard of.

3. Apple cider vinegar. I mentioned in the Introduction how a glass of apple cider vinegar (or ACV for short) diluted in water and a dollop of honey keeps colds and flu at bay. ACV is made from squeezed liquid of crushed apples. Sugar and yeast are added to the liquid to start the fermentation process, which turns the sugar into alcohol. During a second round of fermentation, the alcohol is converted into vinegar by acetic acid-forming bacteria. The acetic acid is what gives vinegar its sour taste.

The acidity in ACV helps the body rebalance its acid level, which is important as the body tries to find its equilibrium after fighting off cold and flu viruses. The icky taste hasn't stopped aficionados from singing the praises of ACV. Remember: don't drink ACV unless it is well diluted. I recommend two to three tablespoons of ACV and one tablespoon of honey mixed in eight to twelve ounces of water.

4. Garlic, onions, and horseradish. You'll have pleasing breath after you mash these three ingredients in a bowl and lick a spoonful. I'm teasing, of course, but I'm serious about the cold-and-flu-fighting capabilities of garlic, onions, and horseradish. Garlic is one of nature's most potent germ fighters, and this pungent bulb will do a spring cleaning if allowed to go after any nasty-minded cold and flu germs in the neighborhood. A summary of garlic research that appeared in the *Physicians' Desk Reference for Herbal Medicine* suggested that garlic improves the activity of natural killer cells, which takes on cancer cells and cold-and-flu viruses that invade the body.[8]

Garlic, onions, and horseradish contain agents that have a chemical resemblance to drugs found in drugstore medications. Known as "hot foods," these ingredients have antimicrobial properties, drying up nasal passages and airways, and reducing mucus buildup.

5. Ginger. This superstar spice deserves its own category. Ginger, the world's most widely cultivated spice, contains natural chemicals that stimulate the production of anti-inflammatory agents like eicosanoids. "Besides reducing fever, historical and modern research shows that ginger is also capable of relieving chills caused by the common cold and warming the body," wrote Paul Schulick, author of *Ginger: Common Spice & Wonder Drug.* Schulick added that ginger tea is the perfect cold remedy because of its antitoxic properties. If the cayenne pepper in the Cold and Flu Bustin' Spicy Chicken Soup recipe doesn't clear your nostrils, then ginger will finish the job![9]

If you feel a cold or flu coming on, pour a cup of boiling water over two tablespoons of freshly grated ginger and let it steep for five to ten minutes. Then add a dash of hot sauce, or the juice of one lemon, and one to two tablespoons of raw honey, depending on your preferred taste. Sip throughout the day.

I'm also high on cayenne pepper, as you can tell. This anti-bacterial is a stimulant that improves circulation. Capsaicin—the chemical that makes cayenne pepper hot—is actually a counterirritant, meaning it's an irritation to an irritation. When you're coughing and battling a bug, this means that cayenne pepper can reduce pain and swelling, and is therefore useful as a topical analgesic. It also stimulates circulation and perspiration, which helps to break up congestion.

Don't go overboard with one of nature's hottest spices: be sure to season lightly since a little too much can set your mouth on fire.

6. Water. After eating any food or chicken soup seasoned with cayenne pepper, you may be reaching for a tall glass of water. Water isn't a food, of course, but this calorie- and sugar-free substance performs many vital tasks for the body: regulating the body temperature, carrying nutrients and oxygen to the cells, cushioning joints, protecting organs and tissue, and removing toxins.

There's another reason why family physicians pat you on the back and remind you to drink plenty of fluids. Water not only helps thin mucus secretions, but it also clears toxins from the respiratory tract and transports them to the liver and kidneys for disposal. Water greatly increases the efficiency of the immune system and is vital because fluids in urine eliminate waste products.

When you're battling a cold or fever, the body needs plenty of water. I think my propensity for staying well hydrated is one reason I don't get slammed by colds or the flu. I sip water throughout the day, setting a forty-eight-ounce bottle of water on my office desk as a reminder to keep putting fluids into my system. My record for drinking water is one and one-quarter gallons of water in a day during a fast, but I won't reveal how many trips I made to the bathroom that day.

Sure, you'll go to the bathroom more often, but is that so bad? Drinking plenty of water is not only healthy for the body, but it's a key part of the Great Physician's Rx for Colds and Flu Battle Plan (see page 75), so keep a water bottle close by and drink water before, during, and in between meals.

This seems a good place to talk about this country's obsession with coffee and tea, thanks to your neighborhood Starbucks. Although coffee and tea have been consumed for thousands of years by some of the world's healthiest people, I don't think it's a good idea to drink coffee when you're battling a cold or flu. Teas and herbal infusions (the latter beverage is made from herbs and spices, rather than the actual tea plant) are a better story all together.

Infusions of herbs and spices such as teas have been a part of nearly every culture throughout history. In fact, consuming organic teas and herbal infusions as you're recuperating from a respiratory illness can be one of the best things you can do for your health. Green and white teas, for example, provide the body with antioxidants such as polyphenols, which help reduce cellular damage and oxidative stress. Studies have identified these compounds as helping to increase metabolism. Teas and herbal infusions can provide energy, enhance the immune system, improve digestion, and even help you wind down after a long day.

My favorite tea blends contain combinations of tea (green, black, or white) with biblical herbs and spices such as grape, pomegranate, hyssop, olive, and fig leaves. Even though I've never thought of myself as a tea-drinking type, my wife, Nicki, and I enjoy these biblical tea blends with dinner.

You'll find in my Great Physician's Rx for Colds and Flu Battle Plan (see page 75) that I recommend a cup of hot tea and honey with breakfast, dinner, and during snack time. I also advise consuming freshly made iced tea, as tea can be consumed hot or steeped and iced. Please note that while herbal tea provides many great health benefits, nothing can replace pure water for hydration.

7. **Cultured dairy products.** Dairy products are said to be mucus producing, so should you eschew dairy when you feel a cold or flu coming on?

Most people who avoid dairy products while battling a respiratory illness generally do so to avoid having more nasal congestion and throat phlegm. Cutting back on dairy, especially products made from cow's milk, makes sense when you're battling a cold or flu. But when you're healthy, I believe in eating cultured dairy products from goats, cows, and sheep. Dairy products derived from goat's milk and sheep's milk can be healthier for some individuals than those from cows, although dairy products from organic or grass-fed cows can be excellent as well, as long as the dairy is non-homogenized.

Goat's milk is less allergenic because it does not contain the same complex proteins found in cow's milk. Goat's milk contains higher amounts of medium-chain fatty acids (MCFAs) than other milks, and contains 7 percent less lactose than cow's milk. It's been said that raw or cultured goat's milk fully digests in a baby's stomach in just twenty minutes, while pasteurized cow's milk can take eight hours. The difference lies in the goat milk's structure: its fat and protein molecules are tiny in size, which allows for rapid absorption in the digestive tract.

I also urge you to consume cultured dairy products, such as yogurt and kefir, which provide an excellent source of easily digestible protein, B vitamins, calcium, and probiotics.

WHAT NOT TO EAT

Whether you're trying to avoid a cold or flu bug or you're recovering from one, here is a list of foods that should never find a way onto your plate or into your hands. I call them "The Deadly Dozen."

1. "Unclean" meats and pork products. I have reasons for recommending that you stay away from meats like bacon and ham lunch meat. In all of my previous books, I've consistently pointed out that pork—America's "other white meat"—should be avoided because pigs were called "unclean" in Leviticus and

Exodus. God created pigs as scavengers—animals that survive just fine on any farm slop, water swill, and animal waste tossed their way. Pigs have a simple stomach arrangement: whatever a pig eats goes down the hatch, straight into the stomach, and out the back door in four hours max. They'll even eat their own excrement, if hungry enough.

Even if you decide to keep eating commercial beef instead of the organic version, I absolutely urge you to stop eating pork. Read Leviticus 11 and Deuteronomy 14 to learn what God said about eating clean versus unclean animals, where Hebrew words used to describe "unclean meats" can be translated as "foul" and "putrid," the same terms the Bible uses to describe human waste.

2. Shellfish and fish without fins and scales, such as catfish, shark, and eel. Am I saying *au revoir* to lobster thermidor and *sayonara* to shrimp tempura? That's what I'm saying.

Shellfish and fish without fins and scales, such as catfish, shark, and eel, are also described in Leviticus 11 and Deuteronomy 14 as "unclean meats." God called hard-shelled crustaceans such as lobster, crab, shrimp, and clams unclean because they are "bottom feeders," content to sustain themselves on excrement from other fish. To be sure, this purifies water but does nothing for the health of their flesh—or yours, if you eat them.

The healthiest meat is fish caught in the wild, including salmon, sardines, herring, mackerel, tuna, snapper, bass, and cod. Fish caught in the wild are a richer source of omega-3 fats, protein, potassium, vitamins, and minerals than "farm-raised" fish, which are raised in cement ponds and fed a diet of food pellets. You can purchase fresh salmon and other wild-caught fish from your local fish market or health food store.

3. Hydrogenated oils. This means margarine and shortening are taboo, as well as any commercial cakes, pastries, desserts, and anything with the words *hydrogenated* or *partially hydrogenated* on the label. Hydrogenated oils contain trans-fatty acids, which can lead to arterial inflammation, one of the major risk factors for heart disease.

4. Artificial sweeteners. Aspartame (found in NutraSweet and Equal), saccharine (Sweet'N Low), and sucralose (Splenda) are chemicals several hundred times sweeter than sugar. In my book, artificial sweeteners should be completely avoided whether they come in blue, pink, or yellow packets.

5. White flour. White flour isn't a problematic chemical like artificial sweeteners, but it's virtually worthless and not healthy for you.

6. White sugar. Since sugar suppresses your immune system and impairs your defenses against infectious disease, this carbohydrate should be severely restricted.

7. Soft drinks. Nothing more than liquefied sugar. A twenty-ounce bottle of Coke or Pepsi is the equivalent of eating fifteen teaspoons of sugar. Diet drinks loaded with artificial sweeteners are even worse.

8. Corn syrup. Another version of sugar and just as bad for you, if not worse.

9. Pasteurized homogenized skimmed milk. Like I said, whole organic, non-homogenized milk is better, and goat's milk is best. To give the immune system a real boost, I recommend cultured dairy products.

10. Hydrolyzed soy protein. Hydrolyzed soy protein is found in imitation meat products such as imitation crab. I would look at hydrolyzed soy protein like I would regard meat cured with nitrites: stay away from it. You're always going to be better off eating organic meats.

11. Artificial flavors and colors. These are never good for you under the best of circumstances, and certainly not when you're battling a cold or flu.

12. Excessive alcohol. Although studies point out the benefits of drinking small amounts of red wine for the heart (part of the "French Paradox"), the fact remains that alcohol contains lots of calories, and wine usually contains lots of sugar, neither of which are good when battling an infection.

EAT: WHAT FOODS ARE EXTRAORDINARY, AVERAGE, OR TROUBLE?

I've prepared a comprehensive list of foods that are ranked in descending order based on their health-giving qualities. Foods at the top of the list are healthier than those at the bottom. The best foods to serve and eat are what I call "Extraordinary," which God created for us to eat and will give you the best chance to live a long and happy life. It's best if at least 75 percent of your diet is made up of foods from the Extraordinary category.

Foods in the Average category should make up less than 25 percent of your daily diet and be consumed sparingly. Foods in the Trouble category should be consumed with extreme caution or avoided completely.

For a complete listing of Extraordinary, Average, and Trouble Foods, visit www.BiblicalHealthInstitute.com and click on "What to E.A.T."

℞ THE GREAT PHYSICIAN'S RX FOR COLDS AND FLU: EAT TO LIVE

- *Eat only foods God created.*

- *Eat foods in a form that is healthy for the body.*

- *Consume liberal amounts of homemade spicy chicken soup.*

- *Consume spices such as garlic, ginger, and horseradish daily.*

- *If you have a fever, it's best to consume lots of fluids and very little food.*

- *Consume foods high in omega-3 fatty acids.*

- *Consume foods high in fiber.*

- *Avoid foods high in sugar.*

- *Avoid foods containing hydrogenated oils.*

Take Action

To learn how to incorporate the principles of eating to live into your daily life, please turn to page 75 for the Great Physician's Rx for Colds and Flu Battle Plan.

KEY #2

Supplement Your Diet with Whole Food Nutritionals, Living Nutrients, and Superfoods

I was born in the mid-1970s, a time when everyone was talking about a book written by Linus Pauling, PhD, a brainy quantum mechanics chemist and the only person to win two unshared Nobel Prizes. Dr. Pauling's revolutionary book, *Vitamin C and the Common Cold,* postulated that taking 1,000 milligrams of vitamin C daily would reduce the incidence of colds by 45 percent for most people. A thousand milligrams (or 1 gram) happened to be a massive amount of vitamin C because the recommended daily allowance (RDA) is 60 mg.[1]

My father, Herb Rubin, a chiropractor and naturopathic doctor, tells me that back in the '70s cold and flu sufferers were gulping vitamin C tablets like kids reaching for a bowl of M&M's. Vitamin C, chemically known as ascorbic acid and found naturally in citrus fruits and juices, strawberries, cantaloupes, broccoli, and red and green peppers, was suddenly a hot commodity. After the mainstream media—*New York Times, Newsweek, Reader's Digest*—jumped on the bandwagon and spread the gospel of vitamin C megatherapy, the idea of downing a handful of vitamin C tablets to stave off a cold became conventional wisdom for the baby-boomer crowd.

Dr. Pauling must have made quite an impression on my parents' generation, because I run into a lot of people who tell me that vitamin C is their go-to supplement at the first sign of a sniffle. Today vitamin C has a reputation for being helpful in the treatment of colds and flu as well as strengthening tissues and promoting wound healing. Ranking among the top five vitamins sold in the U.S. each year, millions start their mornings by knocking back multivitamins with vitamin C or chomping on a couple of orangey-tasting chewable vitamin C tablets.

There's no doubt that the body needs *some* vitamin C on a regular basis to survive: everyone learned in grade school how Christopher Columbus and other explorers to the New World battled scurvy because they didn't eat fresh fruit while they sailed the ocean blue. Then again, no one knew five hundred years ago that vitamin C helps your body resist infection and builds healthy bones, teeth, and gums.

Flash forward to the present day: Was Dr. Pauling correct? Is vitamin C a modern-day cure for the common cold? After all, it's been more than thirty-five years since the so-called "Father of Vitamin C" issued his manifesto, plenty of time for medical researchers to pick up vitamin C by its ankles and give it a good shake or two.

The answer depends on who you listen to. Alternative medicine practitioners say that there are "numerous studies" showing that people who take large doses of vitamin C report reductions in the incidence, severity, and duration of colds, but traditional medicine remains unconvinced.[2] *Encyclopedia of Natural Medicine* sums up this dichotomy, saying, "Since 1970, there have been over twenty double-blind studies designed to test Pauling's assertion. Yet despite the fact that in every study the group that received vitamin C had a decrease either in duration or in severity of symptoms, for some reason the clinical effect is still debated in the medical community."[3]

Encyclopedia of Natural Medicine has that right. The general feeling I get from reading traditional medicine's take is that vitamin C in massive amounts does not prevent colds and at best may slightly reduce the symptoms of a cold, probably as a result of an antihistamine-like effect. Even the Linus Pauling Institute, established on the Oregon State University campus in 1991, feels the same way. (Dr. Pauling died in 1994 after a hale and hearty ninety-three years on earth.) Here's what the official Linus Pauling Institute Web site says about vitamin C and colds:

> The work of Linus Pauling stimulated public interest in the use of large doses (greater than 1 gram/day) of vitamin C to prevent infection with the viruses responsible for the common cold. Reviews of the research conducted on this issue over the past twenty years conclude that, in general, large doses of vitamin C do not have a significant effect on the incidence of the common cold. However, a few studies have indicated that certain susceptible groups (e.g., individuals with low dietary intake and marathoners) may be less susceptible to the common cold when taking supplemental vitamin C. Additionally, large doses of vitamin C have been found to decrease the duration and severity of colds, an effect that may be related to the antihistamine effects found to occur with large doses (2 grams) of vitamin C.[4]

Here's where I come down on taking vitamin C and other supplements for cold and flu symptoms, and I'll express myself through the use of a football metaphor: Pretend that the Cold Warriors have the football and your team is playing defense. The Cold Warriors—those agents trying to score on your body—are constantly attacking, constantly probing your immune system. Most of the time you're able to stop them. On this offensive set of downs, the Cold Warriors are in a third-down-and-long situation, so your team adds an extra pass defender to guard against the long completion.

That's the same idea when it comes to using supplements. When a cold or flu comes charging my way, I go into a defensive mode and take more supplements to give my body the extra defenders it needs to prevent a cold or flu from scoring. Vitamin C happens to be just one of those supplements, but I also think echinacea, zinc, elderberry, goldenseal, and even over-the-counter combination herbal/vitamin/mineral tablets such as Airborne are worthwhile "defenders" against a cold and flu offensive. Let's take a closer look at some of these other nutrients:

Echinacea. I've already described some of the cold-battling qualities attributed to echinacea in the Introduction. It's better to take this herb from the purple coneflower in the early stages of a cold or flu because it is not an antibiotic, meaning that it doesn't kill germs. Also, echinacea stimulates the production of white blood cells, which can speed to the area of infection and do battle with germy invaders.

Zinc. I grew up sucking on zinc lozenges whenever cold symptoms paid a visit. The lozenges release zinc ions into the mouth where they go directly to the infected nasal tissues. Zinc is a crucial nutrient for optimal immune system function. According to research findings reported in *Annals of Internal Medicine*, zinc lozenges shortened cold duration significantly, and Michael Macknin, PhD and coworker at the Cleveland Clinic Foundation, reported that colds lasted only 4.4 days compared with 7.6 days in the placebo group.[5]

Encyclopedia of Natural Medicine reports that not all zinc lozenges are effective, probably due to different formulations. The best zinc lozenges to use contain the amino acid *glycine* as a sweetener instead of agents like sorbitol and mannitol. If you feel a cold coming on, you may find dissolving a zinc lozenge in your mouth every couple of hours to be an effective remedy.

Joe Mercola, an osteopathic physician and founder of the popular Web site Mercola.com says that he's been using zinc lozenges for himself and in his practice for fifteen years with great success. He advises patients to suck—not swallow—their lozenges and that smaller lozenges are better. Caution: if the lozenges make you nauseated, spit 'em out.

Elderberry. This herb from a fragrant, flowering tree contains antioxidant flavonoids that stabilize cell walls against foreign intruders like flu and cold viruses. Teas made from elderberry fruits or flowers have been a folklore treatment for colds and flu for centuries. Researchers believe that elderberry has an ability to stop flu viruses from replicating, which is the end of the ballgame since flu viruses must reproduce in order to infect the body. A study conducted in 2003 showed that elderberry reduced symptoms and shortened the duration of flu in fifty-four participants between the ages of eighteen and fifty-four. On average, these flu patients recovered in 3.1 days, compared to 7.1 days for those given a placebo.[6]

Elderberry is available in powders, capsules, and liquid fruit extract. Taking a liquid extract or tablet preparation is the way most people prefer to use elderberry against a respiratory infection.

Goldenseal. This herb, which grows as a wild plant in moist, mountainous areas of North America, can help relieve the inflammation of mucous membranes and stop cold and flu viruses from multiplying. Goldenseal is said to work well with echinacea, so you might want to consider taking a combination herbal supplement containing goldenseal and echinacea.

Prescription for Nutritional Healing cautions against taking goldenseal on a daily basis for more than a week or using it at all if you are pregnant or nursing.

Airborne. I travel a great deal, and every now and then on a flight, I'll see a passenger drop a dollar-sized tablet into a plastic cup of water and watch it fizz. It's not Alka-Seltzer—although I wouldn't blame some people for taking an antacid after eating an oxymoronic "airline meal"—but a tablet of Airborne.

What is Airborne? If you don't know, then you're behind the cultural curve. In the fall of 2004, Oprah Winfrey invited a second-grade schoolteacher, Victoria Knight-McDowell, to tell the world about this "wonder remedy" she developed after she got fed up with catching colds from her cherubic students. She informed Oprah that for several years she experimented with various vitamins and herbal substances until she discovered a blend of seven herbs that flood the body with amino acids, antioxidants, and electrolytes. (The ingredients on the label are vitamin A, vitamin C, vitamin E, magnesium, zinc, selenium, manganese, and potassium organic herbal extracts: lonicera, forsythia, schizonepeta, ginger, Chinese vitex, isatis root, and echinacea, along with the amino acids glutamine and lysine.)

When Oprah told her audience that she was an Airborne believer and had stocked up on all five flavors, the mega-influential talk show host created a nationwide stampede into Walgreens and Long's Drugs.

Airborne was no longer Victoria's secret.

Okay, a horrible pun, but since then Airborne has enjoyed a cultlike status among the true believers who can't fathom the thought of boarding a passenger jet without bringing a seven-dollar tube of Airborne on board. As soon as the drink cart passes by, they're plopping an effervescent tablet of Airborne into a glass of water.

I've taken Airborne once or twice on a plane flight, but I prefer to practice advanced hygiene whenever I feel a cold or flu coming on after flying cross-country (I'll explain why in the next chapter). Still, I have friends who swear by Airborne, so you just may want to try a plop-fizz the next time you board a flight or begin hacking at home.

WHAT TO TAKE WHEN YOU'RE NOT
BATTLING A COLD OR FLU

Echinacea, zinc, and elderberry are some of the nutrients that I would reach for when I'm battling a cold or flu, but when it comes to viral bugs, the old saying—"An ounce of prevention is worth a pound of cure"—certainly applies here. While I don't believe seasonal colds or flu are totally preventable, I do think that taking nutritional supplements *before* you get sick can reduce the number of colds and flu you experience each season.

Nutritional supplements, living nutritionals, and superfoods are an important part of *The Great Physician's Rx for Colds and Flu.* Topping my list are "whole food" or "living" multivitamins produced from raw materials by adding vitamins and minerals to a living probiotic culture. These vitamins contain different compounds such as organic acids, antioxidants, and key nutrients. They are more costly to produce since the ingredients— fruits, vegetables, sea vegetables, seeds, spices, vitamins and minerals, etc.—are put through a fermentation process similar to the digestive process of the body, but they are well worth the extra money.

The most common form of multivitamins, however, are synthetically produced in a chemist's lab, and are also the cheapest to manufacture. Synthetic vitamins are never going to be as good or potent as ones produced from natural sources; studies show that synthetically made vitamins are 50–70 percent less biologically active than vitamins created from natural sources.

For instance, consider the recommendation to take massive

amounts of vitamin C when you feel a cold coming on. My research into the production of vitamin C shows that synthetically made vitamin C dominates much of the commercial supplement market. What's happened is that vitamin companies have succumbed to market forces that are pushing them to produce vitamin C tablets cheaper than the other guy. For example, you can purchase five hundred 1000-milligram vitamin C tablets from Costco for less then ten bucks. (China has apparently been producing synthetically made vitamin C by the tons.)

Biochemists in white lab coats have peered through their microscopes and figured out ways to synthetically create—although I prefer the verb *imitate*—complex structures such as vitamin C. They do this by synthesizing compounds that may look the same as the nutrients God created in foods. While these isolated nutrients are representative of man's genius inside the laboratory, they are also nutritional folly because they skip the entire process of nature.

The human body was not designed to consume these artificial and unnatural products, especially in the massive amounts that some health professionals advocate. For instance, if you feel a cold coming on and swallow ten 1000-milligram vitamin C tablets during the course of a day, that would be the equivalent of eating 150 oranges. Talk about a colon cleanse! (By the way, one of the side effects of megadoses of vitamin C tablets is diarrhea.)

I think it's unnatural—and physically impossible—to eat 150 oranges in one day, and I don't think God designed us to process ten thousand milligrams of synthetic vitamin C when the flu bug is going around either. I think it's better to consistently take nutritional supplements, living nutrients, and superfoods *before* you get a cold or flu to strengthen your immune system from a viral attack. Here's my "all-star" list:

Whole food multivitamins. If you've taken a gram of vitamin C and a handful of other vitamins, then you've probably noticed that your urine changes to a fluorescent yellow. But the body can't absorb more than 50 percent of the vitamins and minerals you ingest, which means you're receiving only 25 percent of the advertised potency from chemically produced multivitamins.

When you take a whole food natural source multivitamin, however, you'll double the nutrients absorbed by the body. They are more costly to produce since ingredients like antioxidant-rich fruits and vegetables, sea vegetables, and microalgae are put through a fermentation process similar to the digestive process of the body. Whole food multivitamins are well worth the extra money, however.

Omega-3 cod-liver oil complex. One hundred and fifty years ago, if you lived in a fishing community along the coast of Norway, Scotland, or Iceland and came off a boat sneezing up a storm, you couldn't run down to Wal-Mart for some Sudafed or NyQuil. In those days, you were more likely to sip a large spoonful of cod-liver oil.

Cod-liver oil? You mean that horrible-tasting stuff that my grandparents took when they were kids? I sure do, and the reason why seafarers of yesteryear turned to cod-liver oil, which they extracted from the filleted livers of cod, was because they had learned that its medicinal properties were a natural, effective remedy for colds and flu. They didn't know *why* cod-liver oil was good for you; they just knew that it was.

These days, we have a better idea why because of modern science, which has discovered that cod-liver oil contains four nutrients that we hardly get enough of: eicosapentaenoic acid (EPA), docosahexaenoic acid (DHA), vitamin A, and vitamin D.

EPA and DHA are long-chain polyunsaturated fats known as omega-3 fatty acids, which are found in cold-water fish and eggs from chickens that run around and eat worms. When it comes to cold and flu, these omega-3 fatty acids strengthen the immune system so that your colds and flu will be short-lived.

I know that people turn up their runny noses at the thought of sipping a teaspoon of this fishy-smelling liquid, but they shouldn't. These days, cod-liver oil comes in lemon mint and other flavors that mask the odor and taste; for the less daring, omega-3 cod-liver oil comes in easy-to-swallow liquid capsules.

Antioxidants. Fruits, vegetables, herbs, and spices contain a broad array of antioxidants, which are compounds that preserve and protect other compounds in the body from free radical damage. Without going into a long explanation, free radicals are something you don't want to run rampant within your molecular system. Free radicals are oxygen molecules with a single electron, but these unstable molecules are known to attack the immune system's cells. As you know, the immune system gets pummeled by cold and flu germs.

Antioxidants neutralize free radicals, which is a good thing in the fight against the common cold. You can add a fruit blend of antioxidant powder to drink to introduce more antioxidants into your system, as well as take a whole food multivitamin, which contains well-known antioxidants such as vitamins E and C and beta-carotene.

Probiotics. Most people, when they see their family physician for a sinus problem or a nasty bronchitis infection, walk out of the doctor's office holding a prescription for antibiotics. Medically speaking, antibiotics are a variety of natural or synthetic substances that inhibit the growth of—or destroy—microorganisms. Since their discovery in the 1930s, antibiotics have made it possible to cure bacteria-related diseases such as pneumonia, tuberculosis, and meningitis. So if antibiotics are supposed to be good for us, what about probiotics? Does that mean they're bad for us?

Just the opposite, I can assure you. By definition, probiotics are living, direct-fed microbials (DFMs) that promote the growth of beneficial bacteria in the intestines. In fact, I would argue that the lack of probiotics in our diet could be associated with allergies, frequent colds, and the flu. Our society has developed into an antibiotic culture so intent on destroying bacteria that we've eradicated much of the beneficial bacteria in our bodies and the environment.

I believe it's important to reintroduce beneficial bacteria into our bodies through dietary supplements containing probiotics. The best probiotics on the market contain soil-based organisms (SBOs), although you can also find foods containing probiotic bacteria in your grocery store's dairy case, where you can reach for probiotic-rich yogurt, kefir, or raw sauerkraut.

Enzymes. When you eat raw foods such as salads and fruits, you consume the enzymes they contain. When you eat cooked or processed meals, like those you get in a restaurant, however, the body's pancreas must produce the enzymes necessary to digest the meal. The constant demand for enzymes strains the pancreas, which must kick in more enzymes to keep up with the demand. Without receiving the proper levels of enzymes from raw or fermented foods—or from taking supplements—you are susceptible to excessive gas and bloating, constipation, heartburn, and low energy.

How do digestive enzymes relate to colds and flu? A cold or flu is sometimes a friendly reminder that your body needs to eliminate waste and toxins that have accumulated in the bloodstream. That's why doctors urge you to "drink plenty of liquids" at the end of an office visit—they want you to flush out your system. You *need* to eliminate excess waste to get your body running cleanly on all cylinders again. That's why you feel sluggish and out of it when cold and flu symptoms come on—and why the body needs to get rid of unwanted waste.

Digestive enzymes can help in that process. These complex proteins are involved in the digestive process—the body's day laborers, the ones responsible for synthesizing, delivering, and eliminating the unbelievable number of ingredients and chemicals your body uses during the waking hours. If you're battling a cold, take plant-based digestive enzymes to streamline digestion and help your body get rid of built-up toxins. (You can find recommended brands by visiting www.BiblicalHealthInstitute.com and clicking on the GPRx Resource Guide.)

Whole food fiber blend. Consuming adequate fiber ensures a feeling of satiety as fiber delays the absorption of sugars in the body and provides a sense of fullness. Fiber improves regularity, which helps to efficiently eliminate toxins from the body. Unfortunately, most of us get about one-fifth of the optimal amount of fiber in our daily diet, which is why I recommend taking a whole food fiber supplement. Look for one that supplies your body with a highly usable, vegetarian source of dietary fiber.

Be sure to choose a brand made from organic seeds, grains, and legumes that are fermented or sprouted for ease of digestion. One of the best ways to consume whole food fiber is by taking a combination green superfood/fiber blend first thing in the morning and just before bed. Simply mix it with your favorite juice or water, and you're giving your body more nutrition than most people get that day—or perhaps that week. Look for a green food fiber blend containing beta-glucans from soluble oat fiber, which can aid in providing satiety for the body and promoting a healthy body weight. (For a list of recommended whole food fiber products, visit www.BiblicalHealthInstitute.com and click on the GPRx Resource Guide.)

Green superfoods. The dislike of eating vegetables, especially green vegetables, follows many people into adulthood. They know that they *should* eat more vegetables, but they regard salads and vegetable servings as colorful decorations for the main event—the meat and potatoes. Many people feel this way: the United States Department of Agriculture estimates that more than 90 percent of the U.S. population fails to eat the recommended three to five servings of vegetables each day.

You're not eating healthily if you eschew your vegetables, especially the most beneficial—deep green leafy vegetables. I know that fresh veggies can be more difficult to find during the winter months, but purchasing salads, green beans, peas, and broccoli is a wise buy. Be thankful that we have a modern transportation system that delivers fresh salads and vegetables into every nook and cranny of our land, even in the dead of winter. (I'm sure our ancestors are spinning in their graves at how ungrateful we've become regarding this technological miracle.)

There's another way to get your green foods that works great during the cold-and-flu season. It's through the consumption of green superfood powders and caplets, which are an excellent and easy way to receive the vitamins, minerals, antioxidants, and enzymes found in green leafy vegetables. All you do is mix green superfood powder in water or juice, or you can choose to swallow a handful of caplets. (For a list of recommended green food products, visit www.BiblicalHealthInstitute.com and click on the GPRx Resource Guide.)

THE GREAT PHYSICIAN'S RX FOR COLDS AND FLU: SUPPLEMENT YOUR DIET WITH WHOLE FOOD NUTRITIONALS, LIVING NUTRIENTS, AND SUPERFOODS

When you're experiencing symptoms:

- *Consume a botanical herb and spice combination containing echinacea, elderberry, goldenseal, hyssop, garlic, and horseradish with each meal.*

- *Consume a botanical CO_2 extract spice blend morning and evening.*

- *Take a whole food multivitamin / mineral with zinc.*

- *Take one to three tablespoons or three to nine capsules of an omega-3 cod-liver oil complex with dinner.*

For everyday good health and cold and flu prevention:

- *Take a whole food living multivitamin with each meal.*

- *Consume one to three teaspoons or three to nine capsules of omega-3 cod-liver oil per day.*

- *Take a whole food fiber / green food blend with beta-glucans from soluble oat fiber twice per day morning and evening.*

- Take an antioxidant/energy product with vitamin B, folic acid, and chromium with each meal.

- Take enzymes and probiotics with each meal.

Take Action

To learn how to incorporate the principles of supple-
menting your diet with whole food nutritionals, living
nutrients, and superfoods into your daily life, please
turn to page 75 for the Great Physician's Rx for Colds
and Flu Battle Plan.

KEY #3

Practice Advanced Hygiene

Remember the SAT test?

I sure haven't forgotten the ulcer-inducing Saturday morning huddled over a desk, filling in dots with the lead of #2 pencils, racing against time to answer every question. Cogitating that hard for four hours drained me.

To introduce Key #3, I've come up with an SAT-type test to start things off here. Don't worry; there's only one question, so here it goes:

> Select the correct analogy:
>
> Colds and flu are to poor hygiene as:
>
> (a) house is to foundation
> (b) dinner is to dessert
> (c) forest fires are to camp fires
> (d) jet is to airline schedule

Give up? The correct answer is (c) because poor hygiene lights the fire that eventually causes your immune system to blow up, opening the door to the common cold or the seasonal flu to wreak havoc on your body.

It's my belief that poor hygiene habits are the number one cause of colds and flu in this country and why I feel that Key #3,

"Practice Advanced Hygiene," is perhaps the most important chapter in this book. So far I've written five other books in the Great Physician's Rx series—*GPRx for Cancer, GPRx for Weight Loss, GPRx for Diabetes, GPRx for a Healthy Heart,* and *GPRx for Irritable Bowel Syndrome*—but as important as practicing advanced hygiene is to those other health conditions, it will never be as important in those books as it is here.

The practice of advanced hygiene is significant, because it's your best defense against cold and flu germs. I'm not exaggerating when I say that colds and flu start with the hands—not the respiratory system—because the hands and fingernails are the first areas where germs can establish a foothold. Once germs set up camp on your fingertips, it's only a matter of time before you rub your eyes, scratch your nose, stroke your ears, or touch your mouth, which sets the transfer of germs into motion. Once that happens, your body's immune system is under attack as the germs, like soldiers assaulting the beaches of Normandy, invade the portals to your body. Before you can say, "I think I'm coming down with something," your nose runs like the Mississippi, your throat is scratchy as sandpaper, and you're sneezing like a circus clown trying to get a big laugh.

Maybe you haven't paid attention to how easily germs enter the body through the nasal passageway or the corner of the eyes—the tear ducts—when you touch those areas. All of us rub our faces so often that we don't even know we're doing it half the time, but when skin-on-skin or skin-on-membrane contact is made, you transfer a garden variety of bacteria, allergens, environmental toxins, and viruses from one part of the body to another. In medical terms, it's called auto- or self-inoculation of the conjunctiva (the eyes) or nasal mucosa (the nose) with a contaminated finger.

Tiny microbes find the hands and the soft tissue underneath the fingernail areas to be staging areas for their assault on the body's immune system. Thus, it's imperative to keep the fingernails, the membranes of the eyes, and the membranes in the front part of the nasal passageway clean to stave off colds and flu. According to Australian scientist Kenneth Seaton, Ph.D., an estimated 90 percent of the germs hide underneath your fingernails, no matter how short you keep them trimmed.

Dr. Seaton, who's been studying hygiene since the late 1950s, said that the conventional wisdom in medical circles is that colds and influenza are mainly spread by germs and viruses swirling through the air after one has coughed or sneezed in close proximity. Thus, prevention was thought to be almost impossible, because who can protect themselves from airborne exposure? "For years, I struggled to educate and convince the medical establishment that hand transmission is by far the most efficient mechanism for spreading germs and viruses," says Dr. Seaton.[1]

The Australian scientist was convinced that germs were much more likely to be spread by hand-to-hand contact as opposed to airborne exposure. To test his theory, he commenced a research study where ten healthy people were put into a room with ten other people suffering from an active virus. They spent eight hours together with only one caveat—no physical contact.

At the end of the day, the ten healthy people were tested. Only two of them had become infected. Dr. Seaton repeated his study with ten healthy people put into a room with ten sick people, but this time they were allowed physical contact. After eight hours, you can deduce what happened: all ten healthy people were infected after exposure through physical contact. I guess you could say that germs fly 20 percent of the time and stick out their thumbs for a ride 100 percent of the time. The results prompted Dr. Seaton to coin the phrase, "Germs don't fly; they hitchhike."

During the cold and flu season, many people are afraid they are a ticking time bomb: one false step, and they will blow up like a grenade, sending them to their sickbeds. Actually germs don't quite work that way. They overload the immune system through contact of the fingers with the eyes and nose, and this overload is similar to water filling a balloon in the backyard.

Now, does one water drop cause a balloon to break? No, of course not. It is the accumulation of hundreds of thousands, if not millions, of drops that causes the balloon to explode. It's the same for the germs that attack our bodies.

All Hands on Deck

I'm confident that Dr. Seaton's assertions are correct, just as I'm persuaded that the key to infection control is a simple, three-word command: wash your hands. Not to raise anyone's paranoia, but germs are everywhere that people touch their hands: doorknobs, computer keyboards, shopping carts, check-out stands, money and coins, foods prepared by others, and toilets and sinks, to list a few.

But the most common pass of germs from one to another happens during a simple handshake. If you're in the business world or meeting people regularly—or attending a church event—you're shaking hands with friends and acquaintances. Listen, I do my share of book signings and trade shows where I usually shake hands with a couple hundred people. I have no idea what those hands have been touching, but I'm ruefully aware of a Wirthlin study revealing that 26 percent of males zip up and bypass the washbasin after using a public restroom (the figure was 17 percent for females).[2] Yuck!

Since germs are passed like a hot potato from one to another, it's imperative to take key steps to guard yourself against attack, like washing your hands and nails with a quality semisoft soap and dipping your head into a facial solution that cleanses your eyes and nasal passageways.

After shaking hundreds of hands at a book signing or trade show, the first thing I do after returning to my hotel room is wash my hands. I'm well aware that scrubbing my hands isn't enough because of those germs hibernating under and around my fingernails, so I use a special semisoft hand soap. The creamy-type soap, which comes in a white tub and is rich in essential oils, is not directly antibacterial, however. I believe that antibacterial medicines and soaps end up disrupting the delicate balance of microflora necessary for healthy skin.

I start by dipping both hands into the tub and plunging my fingernails into the creamy soap. Then I work the special cream around the tips of my fingers, cuticles, and fingernails for fifteen to thirty seconds. When I'm finished, I lather my hands for fifteen seconds before rinsing them under running water. After my hands are clean, I take another swab of special soap into my hands and wash my face.

Since I'm aware that the most susceptible entry ports for germs are the tear ducts and nasal passageways, I employ a second step of advanced hygiene, which is called a facial dip. I begin by filling my washbasin or a clean, large bowl with warm but not hot water, and then I add regular table salt and two eyedroppers of a mineral-based facial solution into the cloudy water. Then I bend over and dunk my face into the water, opening my eyes several times to allow the cleansing water to flush out the membranes around my eyes. Immediately after, I dive in once again, keeping my eyes closed and my mouth out of the water while I blow bubbles through my nose. I call it "sink snorkeling."

Then I quickly suck a small amount of water into my nose, which does a Roto-Rooter action by scouring out germs that may have been transferred to my nose. If one of my nostrils is partially blocked, I close the open nostril while underwater and slowly inhale to draw the diluted facial solution into the blocked nostril. That maneuver usually unplugs the nostril. Whenever I feel that I'm coming down with a cold or flu, I do the facial wash four to six times that day, and when I wake up the next morning, I'm as good as new. After my sink snorkeling, I towel off and blow my nose into a tissue. I perform advanced hygiene after waking up in the morning and just before going to bed to avoid getting sick, but when I feel like I'm coming down with something, I perform these advanced hygiene steps *five times* a day. I recommend you do the same.

I've been following this advanced hygiene protocol ever since I learned about it ten years ago when I was very sick. Since then, I've been virtually illness free from the usual respiratory illnesses and sinus infections that afflict millions of Americans each day. Practicing advanced hygiene adds three or four minutes to getting ready for work in the morning or going to bed in the evening, but I think that's a small price to pay for not having to deal with the sniffles, a head cold, or worse.

My final two steps of advanced hygiene involve applying very dilute drops of hydrogen peroxide and minerals into my ears for thirty to sixty seconds to cleanse the ear canal and then brushing my teeth with an essential oil-based tooth solution to cleanse my mouth of unhealthy germs.

The ears are important to keep clean too. Back in 1928, Dr. Richard Simmons—not the fitness guru . . . he's not that old—hypothesized that cold and flu germs can sneak into the body through the ear canal. Dr. Mercola of Mercola.com advises administering a few drops of 3 percent hydrogen peroxide (H_2O_2) into each ear when cold and flu symptoms present themselves. There may be some bubbling or mild stinging in the ear canal, but hydrogen peroxide seems to loosen up ears packed with wax, and its powerful oxidizing qualities kill bacteria and viruses. (Hydrogen peroxide is also a household antiseptic used on cuts and scrapes.)

Finally, there's a protein floating around in your bloodstream that you should know about, and it happens to be the most abundant one. It's called albumin, and this protein transports hormones and nutrients in your bloodstream and moves waste out. Like dump trucks on their way to the landfill, albumin hauls wastes and toxic cells to the liver for degradation and elimination from the body.

Your risk of catching a cold or flu shoots way up when albumin levels in the blood go down. Dr. Seaton is certain that poor hygienic habits cause albumin levels to drop because the immune system can't produce enough to defend the body when under attack by cold and flu viruses. Albumin levels can be optimized by practicing advanced hygiene, which underscores the importance of this key as part of *The Great Physician's Rx for Colds and Flu.*

WORK ENVIRONMENT

I work in a business park in West Palm Beach, Florida, that resembles thousands of others that have sprouted up like spring mushrooms around the country. Today's workplace conditions—I'm thinking of suburban industrial parks filled with stout concrete buildings and warrens of cubicles—are a breeding ground for germs. The trouble is that when employees come down with a cold or flu, they're just as apt to come to work—where they spread their germs to unsuspecting coworkers—than call in sick.

During the cold-and-flu season, I wash my hands every hour or two with special semisoft cream hand soap that I keep at my office. Wiping down your desk with disinfectant once a morning and once an afternoon is another idea. I probably wouldn't go out of my way to shake hands with coworkers who are exhibiting symptoms. And if someone who is clearly sick—constantly sneezing with a nose running like a faucet—I would drop a hint about taking a sick day. If you feel it's not your place to confront a sick employee, call human resources.

You might also tell your human resources director about a survey conducted by Chuck Gerba, a University of Arizona environmental-microbiology professor. "Dr. Germ," as his colleagues call him, found that germs love to lurk in office environments. His researchers tested samples from 328 surfaces—from cubicles to conference rooms—in office buildings around the country and found that microbes causing respiratory infections like bronchiolitis and pneumonia can live on desktops and office surfaces for up to *three* days. They also found viruses and bacteria on telephones, door handles, and light switches. Yuck again![3]

To be forewarned is to be forearmed. If you're going to stave off colds or the flu, particular attention must be paid to practicing advanced hygiene, because colds and flu are gifts that keep on giving.

℞ THE GREAT PHYSICIAN'S RX FOR COLDS AND FLU: PRACTICE ADVANCED HYGIENE

- *Dig your fingers into a semisoft soap with essential oils and wash your hands several times a day during the cold-and-flu season, paying special attention to removing germs from underneath your fingernails.*

- *Cleanse your nasal passageways and the mucous membranes of the eyes daily by performing a facial dip.*

- *Cleanse the ear canals several times per week.*

- *Use an essential oil-based tooth solution daily to remove germs from the teeth, gums, and mouth.*

Take Action

To learn how to incorporate the principles of practicing advanced hygiene in your daily life, please turn to page 75 for the Great Physician's Rx for Colds and Flu Battle Plan.

KEY #4

Condition Your Body
with Exercise and Body Therapies

When's the last time you exercised?

Slept eight hours?

Did absolutely nothing on a Sunday afternoon?

Final question: Had a cold or flu lately?

Listen: I ask myself these questions too. I know that exercise is an important "body therapy" that boosts the immune system and primes the body to resist cold and flu germs. Physical fitness is essential to good health and is one of the best things you can do for your body, mind, and spirit.

Physically active people are less likely to catch a cold, according to a University of South Carolina study of 550 healthy men and women with an average age of forty-eight. The findings showed that those who exercised moderately averaged one cold per year versus the couch potatoes who reported four colds a year.[1]

To me, this is a common-sense confirmation that those who engage in regular physical activity won't be as susceptible to a bug as those who lead sedentary lives. Exercise does a body good: pumping those legs and arms speeds up the heart and makes you breathe faster, which helps transfer oxygen from your lungs to your blood and increase the body's natural virus-killing cells. Exercise stimulates the disease-fighting white blood cells in the body to move from the organs into the bloodstream, where it can mount a defense against those germs that enter the body's portals.

The point of this chapter is that regular exercise—twenty to thirty minutes a day for at least five days a week—can prevent colds and flu. My favorite way to get the body moving is called *functional fitness*, a form of gentle exercise that raises the heartbeat, strengthens the body's core muscles, and exercises the cardiovascular system through the performance of real-life activities in real-life positions.

Functional fitness can be done by using body weight only or by employing dumbbells, mini-trampolines, and stability balls. You can find functional fitness classes and equipment at gyms around the country, including LA Fitness, Bally Total Fitness, and local YMCAs. You'll be asked to perform squats with feet apart, feet together, and one back with the other forward. What you *won't* be asked to perform are high-impact exercises like those found in pulsating aerobics classes. (For more information on functional fitness, visit www.GreatPhysiciansRx.com.)

Walking is another form of gentle exercise that requires no expensive outlay of cash. You can walk whenever it fits into your schedule: the crack of dawn before work, during the morning break, over the lunch hour, before dinner, or in the twilight hours. You can go at your own pace, and, since strength and size don't count for much when it comes to walking, it's a form of exercise you can do with someone of the opposite sex.

Can you—or should you—exercise when you're battling a

cold or flu? If you feel up to it, there's nothing harmful to breaking a sweat, and I've always felt that exercise releases built-up toxins in the body. Moving around loosens up mucus and fluids that build up in the upper respiratory tract, so unless you have a fever, a moderate workout should make you feel better. If you've been hit with a bad flu bug and don't feel like getting out of bed, however, take that as your cue to stay under the covers and eat my homemade spicy chicken soup. (Sorry, I had to get that plug in there again.)

GET SOME REST

You know how family physicians say to drink plenty of fluids and "get some rest"? People somehow pass over that last part.

Listen, I plead guilty as charged. There are days when I'm scheduled to speak at three Sunday morning services at a large church and my nose is running and I'm battling a head cold. I have to power through it, right? But I also know, sooner or later, I'm going to need some downtime.

Going through life without adequate rest happens to millions because sleep is a body therapy in short supply these days. A nationwide "sleep deficit" means that we're packing in as much as we can from the moment we wake up until we crawl into bed sixteen, seventeen, or eighteen exhausting hours later. American adults are down to a little less than seven hours of sleep each night, a good two hours less than our great-great-grandparents slept a hundred years ago.

As for getting enough sleep, again I plead guilty as charged.

Nicki and I are parents of an energetic toddler who wakes us up at 5:30 a.m. on the dot each day. If I happen to go to bed really late, say around 2:00 a.m., I just don't feel well for a couple of days. My tired body is more susceptible to catching a cold or flu bug. When I get to bed before 11:00 p.m., however, I feel better and perform better the next day. I urge you to go to bed earlier, even if it's thirty minutes before you typically go to bed. If you're used to watching Leno or Letterman after you crawl into bed, tape or TiVo the shows for viewing the next day.

Eight hours of sleep is the magic number to shoot for, say the sleep experts. That's because when people are allowed to sleep as much as they would like in a controlled setting, like in a sleep laboratory, they naturally sleep eight hours in a twenty-four-hour time period. This twenty-four-hour period, called the circadian rhythm, mirrors the twenty-four hours it takes for the earth to rotate on its axis as it circles the sun.

HERE COMES THE SUN

Speaking of the sun, there's a correlation between sunning yourself and staying cold free. When your face or your arms and legs are exposed to sunlight, your skin synthesizes vitamin D from the ultraviolet rays of sunlight. The body needs vitamin D, which is not a vitamin but actually a critical hormone that helps regulate the health of more than thirty different tissues and organs, including the lungs. I recommend intentionally exposing yourself to at least fifteen minutes of sunlight a day to increase vitamin D levels in the body.

HYDROTHERAPIES TO THE RESCUE

Nicki and I are fortunate to have a sauna inside our home, and when either of us starts sniffling, inside the sauna we go. Something about sweating profusely and drinking a lot of liquids makes sense when it comes to eliminating viral bugs from the body. Some say that the temperature inside a sauna is too hot for the cold and flu viruses to survive. Sitting in a toasty sauna or taking a steam bath are forms of hydrotherapy that are beneficial against colds and flu. There are also other forms of hydrotherapy—baths, showers, washing, and wraps—that use hot *and* cold water.

For instance, I wake up with a hot shower in the mornings, but then I turn off the hot water and stand under the brisk cold water for about a minute, which totally invigorates me. Cold water stimulates the body and boosts oxygen use in the cells, while hot water dilates blood vessels, which improves blood circulation and transports more oxygen to the brain.

Finally, there's one more body therapy that's part of the Great Physician's prescription for colds and flu. Aromatherapy involves the sense of smell and the use of essential oils in a variety of healing ways. I believe extensive health benefits can be derived from introducing essential oils into your daily regimen. You may add just an eyedropper of essential oils into hot bathwater, burn them in a diffuser, or rub a few drops on your fingers, cup your hands over your mouth and nose, and inhale a deep breath.

The Prescription for Nutritional Healing points out that eucalyptus oil is helpful for relieving congestion.[2] Draw a hot bath, add five drops of eucalyptus oil, and give yourself a good soak. You can also add rosemary and sage oils for good measure.

If you don't want to go to the trouble of taking a bath (or if you don't have a bathtub at home), then you can put six drops of an essential oil blend in two cups of boiling water and inhale the steam. You do this by removing the pot of boiling water from the stove, placing a towel over your head, and inhaling deeply for three to five minutes. Be careful to not get so close to the steam that you burn yourself.

℞ THE GREAT PHYSICIAN'S RX FOR COLDS AND FLU: CONDITION YOUR BODY WITH EXERCISE AND BODY THERAPIES

- *Make a commitment and an appointment to exercise five times a week or more for twenty to thirty minutes, when healthy, to boost the immune system and prevent colds and flu.*

- *Incorporate five to fifteen minutes of functional fitness into your daily schedule.*

- *Practice deep-breathing exercises when you feel a cold or flu coming on. Inflate your lungs to full and hold for several seconds before slowly exhaling.*

- *Go to bed earlier, paying close attention to how much sleep you get before midnight. Do your best to get eight hours of sleep nightly. Remember that sleep is the most important nonnutrient you can incorporate into your health regimen.*

- *End your next shower by changing the water temperature to cool (or cold) and standing underneath the spray for one minute.*

- *During your next break from work, sit outside in a chair and face the sun. Soak up the rays for ten or fifteen minutes.*

- *Use essential oils like eucalyptus to ease nasal congestion.*

Take Action

To learn how to incorporate the principles of conditioning your body with exercise and body therapies into your daily life, please turn to page 75 for the Great Physician's Rx for Colds and Flu Battle Plan.

KEY #5

Reduce Toxins in Your Environment

When I come down with a cold, I usually backtrack the last twenty-four hours to figure out why a bug bested my immune system. Although I can never be sure, I can usually trace a cold to a long plane flight, although a lack of sleep or no exercise can be factors as well.

I know the reason I still get colds isn't because I don't follow the first three Keys of the Great Physician's prescription. I eat an organic diet comprised of foods that God created in a form healthy for the body. As for nutritional supplements, I have a Cal Ripken-like streak going—I haven't missed a day in ten years. And you read in Key #3 how I practice advanced hygiene religiously.

But when it comes to Key #5—"Reduce Toxins in Your Environment"—here's a situation where I'm definitely more vulnerable to catching a sinus bug. Take plane flights, for example. I *know* that parking my body in a cramped coach seat inside the fuselage of a single-aisle Boeing 737 with 137 other coughing, wheezing, and sneezing passengers is doing a number on my immune system. The air in a modern jetliner is a mixture of fresh outside air and gunky recirculated air; a Boeing 737 recirculates about 40 percent of its air, while a 757 recirculates about 50 percent.[1] As far as I'm concerned, recirculated air translates into recirculated germs.

Am I more susceptible to being infected by a cold or flu bug while taking a jet flight? I did some research, and to my surprise, the *Journal of the American Medical Association* (*JAMA*) reported on a study showing that there is *no* evidence that aircraft cabins with recirculated air increases the risk of upper respiratory tract infections (URIs).[2] I guess I should tell those folks sitting in 20D and E that they're wasting their time and money taking Airborne.

But then I read the *JAMA* study more closely, and I began to feel better. Or maybe I mean worse. During the summer of 1999, the study gave questionnaires to 1,100 passengers flying between San Francisco and Denver. Here's the kicker: the study's main point was that those who travel in planes with *recirculated* air are no more likely to catch colds than travelers flying on aircrafts that pump in only *fresh air*.

Time out! I would estimate that 99.9 percent of the flying public flies in planes with recirculated air since the Boeing 727—a '60s-era model—was the last jet constructed to provide 100 percent fresh air to its passengers. Boeing and Airbus construct planes with recirculation air systems as a fuel-saving measure. But get this: the *JAMA* study showed that passengers get far more colds after flights than when they don't fly, and they also get more colds than people who do not fly. So my instincts were right after all. Whenever my schedule requires airline travel—which is virtually every week—I practice advanced hygiene before and after the flight by applying an essential oil blend to my shirt. During my flight, I'll rub the essential oil blend into my hands and then cup my hands and breathe in the oils.

Airline flights aren't the only place where you breathe recirculated air. Care to guess two other prominent places? Your home and your place of work. Anytime you're breathing air-conditioned air, you're breathing recirculated air. In hot areas of the country like Florida, we breathe recirculated air around the clock. The American Lung Association estimates that we spend 90 percent of our time indoors, and that sounds right to me.

According to the U.S. Environmental Protection Agency, which reported the results of a five-year study that surveyed six hundred homes in six cities, peak concentrations of twenty toxic compounds were two hundred to five hundred times higher inside homes than outdoors. Today's well-insulated homes and energy-efficient doors and windows are doing too good a job, trapping "used" air filled with harmful airborne toxins that cause health problems such as colds and flu. That's another reason why colds are more common in winter: people spend more time indoors in close proximity to each other. Ventilation is less efficient, increasing the infection risk as well.

Two things can help. One, open your doors and windows a couple of times a day. It's important to air out the house periodically, no matter how warm or cold the temperature is outside. Changing your air-conditioning and heater filters more often can help, but an even better idea is purchasing a good air filter that can scrub the air, so to speak, of airborne germs. My wife, Nicki, and I have set up four photocatalytic air-treatment systems in our home.

I also have a Pionair air filter inside my office, so that's something you should consider investing in since there isn't anything else you can do about breathing in recirculated air at work except to take periodic "fresh air" breaks.

WHAT TO DRINK

I've already touted the healthy benefits of drinking plenty of fluids when you're battling a cold, but when it comes to reducing toxins in your environment, water is especially important because of its ability to flush out toxins and other metabolic wastes from the body. Water is essential to helping your body fight illness, because your immune system cannot function properly unless you're well hydrated. If you have a fever, it's important to be hydrated because a fever can dry up the body's fluids.

Increasing your intake of water will abate cold- and flu-related headaches and speed up the body's ability to assimilate nutrients from the foods—chicken soup?—you eat and the nutritional supplements you take. Since water is the primary resource for carrying nutrients throughout the body, a lack of adequate hydration results in metabolic wastes assaulting your body—and your immune system. That's why the importance of drinking enough water cannot be overstated when it comes to colds and flu.

Notice that my focus is on water, not on regular or diet soft drinks or beverages such as coffee, tea, and fruit juice, even though the latter can be healthy for you when you're cold free. Regular soft drinks contain gobs of sugar, and diet drinks contain artificial sweeteners like aspartame, acesulfame K, or sucralose. Even though the Food and Drug Administration has approved the use of artificial sweeteners in drinks (and food), these chemical food additives may prove to be detrimental to your health, in my opinion, because we just don't know the long-term impact.

And if you're thinking that energy drinks like Red Bull and SoBe Adrenaline Rush would be good "pick-me-uppers" when you have a cold, then let me remind you that these drinks come "fortified" with caffeine and unhealthy additives. Nothing beats plain old water—a liquid created by God to be totally compatible with your body. You should be drinking the proverbial eight glasses of water daily, whether you have a cold or not.

I don't recommend drinking water straight from the tap, however. Nearly all municipal water is routinely treated with chlorine or chloramine, potent bacteria-killing chemicals. I've installed a whole-house filtration system that removes the chlorine and other impurities out of the water *before* it enters our household pipes. Nicki and I can confidently turn on the tap and enjoy the health benefits of chlorine-free water for drinking, cooking, and bathing. Since our water doesn't have a chemical aftertaste, we're more apt to drink it. A much cheaper alternative is installing inexpensive water filters at your kitchen sink or purchasing a countertop water pitcher with a built in carbon-based filter for less than twenty dollars.

TOXINS ELSEWHERE IN YOUR ENVIRONMENT

There are other toxins not directly related to colds and flu but are important enough to mention because they tax your immune system, leaving you more vulnerable to unhealthy germs:

Plastics. Although I drink bottled water from plastic containers when I'm not at home, I think it's safer to drink water from glass cups because of the presence of dioxins and phthalates added in the manufacturing process of plastic.

Household cleaners. Many of today's commercial house cleaners contain potentially harmful chemicals and solvents that expose people to VOCs—volatile organic compounds—which can cause eye, nose, and throat irritation.

Nicki and I have found that natural ingredients like vinegar, lemon juice, and baking soda are excellent substances that make our home spic-and-span. Natural cleaning products that aren't harsh, abrasive, or potentially dangerous to your family are available in grocery and natural food stores.

Skin care and body care products. Toxic chemicals such as chemical solvents and phthalates are found in lipstick, lip gloss, lip conditioner, hair coloring, hair spray, shampoo, and soap. Ladies, when you rub a tube of lipstick across your lips, your skin readily absorbs these toxins, and that's unhealthy. As with the case regarding household cleaners, you can find natural cosmetics in progressive natural food markets, although they are becoming more widely available in drugstores and beauty stores.

Toothpaste. A tube of toothpaste contains a warning that in case of accidental swallowing, you should contact the local Poison

Control Center. What's that all about? Most commercially available toothpastes contain artificial sweeteners, potassium nitrate, sodium fluoride, and a whole bunch of long, unpronounceable words. Again, search out a healthy, natural version.

℞ THE GREAT PHYSICIAN'S RX FOR COLDS AND FLU: REDUCE TOXINS IN YOUR ENVIRONMENT

- *Pay attention to the amount of airborne germs and microbes—inside and outside your home—especially during the cold-and-flu season.*

- *Improve indoor air quality by opening windows and buying an air-filtration system.*

- *Drink the recommended eight or more glasses of purified water daily—whether you're sick or not.*

- *Use natural cleaning products for your home.*

- *Use natural products for skin care, body care, hair care, cosmetics, and toothpaste.*

Take Action

To learn how to incorporate the principles of reducing toxins in your environment into your daily life, please turn to page 75 for the Great Physician's Rx for Colds and Flu Battle Plan.

KEY #6

Avoid Deadly Emotions

F eeling stressed out?

Better keep a soft pack of Kleenex handy.

Stress is a deadly emotion that researchers have directly and scientifically linked to one's vulnerability to catching a cold or flu. "Although some people may be naturally more susceptible to the common cold than average, a growing body of evidence suggested that the ease with which we are infected is directly related to the amount of stress in our lives," said a *Psychology Today* report. "People who endure large amounts of long-term stress are more likely to become infected with a cold or flu, and suffer more from cold and flu symptoms."[1]

David Skoner, MD, chief of allergy and immunology at Children's Hospital in Pittsburgh, studied the effects of chronic stress on susceptibility to cold and flu infections. "We've found that people who experience more stress are more likely to get sick and experience worse symptoms," he said.[2]

Stress runs down your immune system like a car's battery when the lights have been left on all night, and everyone hit by stress handles it differently. Some flip out when their favorite soap is interrupted because of a late-breaking news event; others can handle serious business setbacks with aplomb. A lot depends on how God wired you to manage stress.

Stress isn't the only deadly emotion on the block: researchers have also identified anger, acrimony, apprehension, agitation, anxiety, and alarm as deadly emotions, and when you experience any of these feelings—whether justified or not—the efficiency of your immune system decreases noticeably for six hours. When frustrated people harbor resentment and unforgiveness, nurse grudges, or seek revenge, their overstimulated bodies produce the same toxins they would have if they had binged on the worst junk food.

Unless your attitude changes, you will become an unhealthy individual literally overnight. Deadly emotions alter the chemistry of your body, and unchecked emotions can be a pervasive force in determining your daily behavior. Eating while under stress causes the liver's bile tubes to narrow, which blocks bile from reaching the small intestine, where food is waiting to be digested. This is not healthy for the body. An old proverb states it well: "What you are eating is not nearly as important as what's eating you."

A positive attitude about life brings fewer cold symptoms, according to Sheldon Cohen, Ph.D., a psychology professor at Carnegie Mellon University. Dr. Cohen and his team interviewed 334 volunteers three evenings a week for two weeks to assess their mental state. The psychologists looked for signs of well-being, vigor, and calm as well as negative feelings like depression, anxiety, and hostility.

The volunteers were then given a squirt of rhinovirus—the germ behind the common cold—up the nose. Then they were medically observed for five days to see what cold symptoms presented themselves. Those with a positive view of life showed fewer signs of being under the weather, according to Dr. Cohen.[3]

Learn to Let Go and to Forgive

If feelings of anger or hostility are welling up inside you, it's probably because someone has said something that was mean-spirited or belittled you. Trust me: I know words can hurt, and words can break a heart.

This is not the time to fall off the healthy food wagon or revert to eating fat-filled and high-sugar "comfort foods" sure to weaken your immune system. This is the time to forgive those who've made your life miserable, made cutting remarks about you or your children, or done something to hurt your family financially.

If you've been hurt in the past by mean-spirited comments and people, I'm sure I'm not the first to urge you to put the past in the rearview mirror and move forward. But you must. If you follow the Great Physician's prescription for a healthy lifestyle, I'm confident that this will help you deal with any deadly emotions weighing on your mind. Please remember that no matter how bad you've been hurt in the past, it's still possible to forgive. "For if you forgive men their trespasses, your heavenly Father will also forgive you," Jesus said says in Matthew 6. "But if you do not forgive men their trespasses, neither will your Father forgive your trespasses" (Matthew 6:14–15).

Forgive those who've hurt you and then let it go. Then memorize this wise advice from King Solomon in the old King James Version: "A merry heart doeth good like a medicine" (Proverbs 17:22 KJV).

℞ THE GREAT PHYSICIAN'S RX FOR COLDS AND FLU: AVOID DEADLY EMOTIONS

- *Realize that you're susceptible to getting sick when you're sad, scared, or stressed by everyday life.*

- *Trust God when you face circumstances that cause you to worry or become anxious.*

- *Practice forgiveness every day and forgive those who hurt you.*

Take Action

To learn how to incorporate the principles of avoiding deadly emotions into your daily life, please turn to page 75 for the Great Physician's Rx for Colds and Flu Battle Plan.

KEY #7

Live a Life of Prayer and Purpose

While surfing the Net, this headline caught my eye:

Nation's Leading Alarmists Excited About Bird Flu

Excited? I have to read more, I thought, so I scrolled through the story's lead paragraphs:

(Washington, D.C.) The avian influenza virus, a mutant flu strain that has claimed the lives of thirty-one people in Eastern Asia since it was first observed passing from birds to humans in 1997, has the nation's foremost alarmists extremely agitated.

"Right now, the bird flu is just a blip in the newspapers, but if the avian influenza virus undergoes antigenic shift with a human influenza virus, the resulting subtype could be highly contagious and highly lethal in humans," Matthew Wexler, the president of the National Alarmist Council and one of the nation's leading fear mongers, said Monday. "My professional opinion, and more importantly, my personal belief, is that this is a cause for great national alarm."

Wexler's sentiments were unanimously upheld by members of the alarmist community.

"The bird flu could cause a global influenza pandemic similar to the Spanish Flu that killed more than 20 million people in 1918," medical alarmist Dr. Preston Douglas said. "Many experts also believe a major global flu outbreak to be immi-nent, if not—God forbid—already underway. Why, recent observation and documentation has recorded at least one case of human-to-human transmission of a rare strain of the avian influenza virus. If this one case is proof that the animal virus is mutating into a contagious, lethal human virus, then the entire world is basically doomed. Doomed!"

Douglas is best known for his brilliant alarmist analyses of flesh-eating bacteria, Ebola, and SARS—all of which he success-fully developed into topics of major international trepidation.[1]

Then I realized I had been had—the "fake news" story was published on The Onion Web site, a satiric online magazine similar to Jon Stewart's *The Daily Show* found weekday evenings on the cable channel, Comedy Central.

Fortunately, bird flu didn't morph into a global epidemic during the winter of 2005–06. If, God forbid, things ever did turn *serious*, I'm thankful that God is bigger than any bird flu epidemic and that He listens to each and every prayer we direct His way.

Start a Small Group

If you have friends or family members struggling with nagging colds or flu that just can't seem to kick, ask them to join you in following the Great Physician's Rx 7 Weeks of Wellness small group study. To learn about joining an existing group in the area or leading a small group in your church, please visit www.GreatPhysiciansRx.com.

Prayer is the foundation of a healthy life, linking your mind, body, and spirit to God. Prayer is two-way communication with our Creator, the God of the universe. There's power in prayer: "The prayer offered in faith will make the sick person well," says James 5:15 NIV.

Prayer is how we talk to God and how He talks to us. There is no greater source of power than talking to the One who made us. Prayer is not a formality; it is not about religion. Prayer is about a relationship—the hotline to heaven. We can talk to God anytime, anywhere, for any reason. He is always there to listen, and He always has our best interests at heart, because we are His children. There was something about facing my mortality back in my college days that made prayer seem very real to me. When my health spun out of control and tumbled into a free fall, I didn't have much else to hang on to but the Lord. In my darkest hour, I spoke with Him constantly.

At times I felt as if I heard God's voice in reply, while on other occasions, He directed me to Scriptures that seemed particularly relevant to my dire situation. What God was teaching me was to listen to Him. Jesus said, "My sheep listen to my voice" (John 10:27 NIV), and I count myself among His flock. Another Scripture seemed particularly apt for my situation: "Blessed is the man who listens to me, watching daily at my doors, waiting at my doorway. For whoever finds me finds life and receives favor from the LORD" (Proverbs 8:34–35). Sometimes when I prayed, the Lord put things on my heart that I hadn't even thought about before I started. Sometimes He didn't answer my prayers in the way I expected Him to, but He transformed my heart to align with His.

In living a healthy, purpose-filled life, prayer is the most powerful tool we possess. Through prayer, God takes away our guilt, shame, bitterness, and anger and gives us a brand-new start. We can eat organic whole foods, supplement our diet with whole food supplements, practice advanced hygiene, reduce toxins, and exercise, but if the spirit is not where it needs to be with God, then we will never be completely healthy. Talking to our Maker through prayer is the foundation for optimal health and makes us whole. After all, God's love and grace are our greatest foods for mind, body, and spirit.

The seventh key to unlocking your health potential is living a life of prayer and purpose. Prayer will confirm your purpose, and it will give you the perseverance to complete it. Seal all that you do with the power of prayer, and watch your life become more than you ever thought possible.

FINDING HIS PURPOSE

"Living a life of purpose" is a buzz phrase these days because of a certain book you've probably read or heard about—*The Purpose-Driven Life* by Rick Warren, pastor of Saddleback Church in Lake Forest, California.

When God took me through two years of horrible sickness before restoring my health, I came out of that experience knowing what my purpose was in life: sharing God's message of health and hope so that people wouldn't have to go through what I did. Everything else that I do today is icing—made with raw honey, of course—on the cake. I can't wait to get up in the morning, hoping that I have the privilege of communicating life-changing principles of good health with one person, one thousand people, or even millions that day through television.

If you say to yourself, *I'm not sure I have a purpose*, you would be wrong. If there is breath in your lungs, you have a purpose; it's ingrained in your being. If you haven't found your purpose yet, search your heart. What makes you feel alive? What are you passionate about? The joys of family? The arts? Teaching others? Your purpose is waiting to be discovered. Pinpoint your passions, and you'll uncover your purpose. Keep in mind that God gives us different desires, different dreams, and different talents for a reason because we are all part of one body. Having a purpose will give you something to live for.

Don't let the common cold or a nasty flu virus keep you down for long. Follow the Great Physician's prescription for colds and flu today and you can bounce back. You can be back on your feet in no time, ready to minister to your family, your loved ones, and your work colleagues.

I've yet to meet anyone who went through the cold-and-flu season saying, "Shucks, when am I going to get sick?"

And I've yet to meet anyone who regretted feeling well and becoming healthier, and you won't either.

℞ THE GREAT PHYSICIAN'S RX FOR COLDS AND FLU: LIVE A LIFE OF PRAYER AND PURPOSE

- *Pray continually.*

- *Confess God's promises upon waking and before going to bed.*

- *Find God's purpose for your life and live it.*

- *Be an agent of change in your life by adopting the 7 Keys into your life.*

Take Action

To learn how to incorporate the principles of living a life of prayer and purpose into your daily life, please turn to page 75 for the Great Physician's Rx for Colds and Flu Battle Plan.

THE GREAT PHYSICIAN'S RX FOR COLDS AND FLU BATTLE PLAN

Please note: The GPRx Battle Plan calls for eating a lot of chicken soup, so I'm reprinting the following recipe, which can be found in Key #1, "Eat to Live." If you have a fever, it is best to consume only chicken soup and plenty of additional fluids (pure water) until the fever is under control.

COLD AND FLU BUSTIN' SPICY CHICKEN SOUP

Ingredients:
1 whole chicken (free range, pastured, or organic)
2–4 chicken feet (optional)
3–4 quarts cold filtered water
1 tablespoon raw apple cider vinegar
4 medium-sized onions, coarsely chopped
8 carrots, peeled and coarsely chopped
6 celery stalks, coarsely chopped
2–4 zucchinis, chopped
4–6 tablespoons extra virgin coconut oil
1 bunch parsley
5 garlic cloves
4 inches grated ginger
2–4 tablespoons Celtic Sea Salt
1/4–1/2 teaspoon cayenne pepper

Directions: If you are using a whole chicken, remove fat glands and the gizzards from the cavity. By all means, use chicken feet if you can find them. Place chicken or chicken pieces in a large stainless steel pot with the water, vinegar, and all vegetables except parsley. Let stand for ten minutes before heating. Bring to a boil and remove scum that rises to the top. Cover and cook for twelve to twenty-four hours. The longer you cook the stock, the more healing it will be. About fifteen minutes before finishing the stock, add parsley. This will impart additional mineral ions to the broth. Remove from heat and take out the chicken and the chicken feet. Let it cool and remove chicken meat from the carcass, discarding the bones and the feet. Drop the meat back into the soup.

DAY 1

Please note: This seven-day plan is designed for those who have cold or flu symptoms. For a daily plan to support immune system health overall, visit www.GreatPhysiciansRx.com.

Upon Waking

Prayer: thank God because this is the day that the Lord has made. Rejoice and be glad in it. Thank Him for the breath in your lungs and the life in your body. Ask the Lord to heal your body. Read Matthew 6:9–13 out loud.

Advanced hygiene (you may practice advanced hygiene up to five times per day when you're battling a cold or flu): for hands and nails, jab fingers into semisoft soap four or five times, and lather hands with soap for fifteen seconds, rubbing soap over cuticles and rinsing under water as warm as you can stand. Take another swab of semisoft soap into your hands and wash your face. Next, fill basin or sink with water as warm as you can stand, and add one to three tablespoons of table salt and one to three eyedroppers of iodine-based mineral solution. Dunk face into water and open eyes, blinking repeatedly underwater. Keep eyes open underwater for three seconds. After cleaning your eyes, put your face back in the water, and close your mouth while blowing bubbles out of your nose. Come up from the water, and then immerse your face in the water once again, gently taking water into your nostrils and expelling bubbles. Come up from the water, and blow your nose into facial tissue. To cleanse the ears, use hydrogen peroxide and mineral-based ear drops, putting two or three drops into each ear and letting stand for sixty seconds. Tilt your head to expel the drops. For the teeth, apply two or three drops of essential oil-based tooth drops to the toothbrush. This can be used to brush your teeth or added to existing toothpaste. After brushing your teeth, brush your tongue for fifteen seconds. (For recommended advanced hygiene products, visit www.BiblicalHealthInstitute.com and click on the GPRx Resource Guide.)

Supplements: drink a mixture of two-to-three tablespoons of organic, unfiltered apple cider vinegar and one tablespoon of raw organic honey mixed in eight ounces of warm water. Take three-to-six caplets of a botanical herb and spice combination with garlic, ginger, elderberry, and echinacea (for recommended products, visit www.BiblicalHealthInstitute.com and click on the GPRx Resource Guide) with eight-to-twelve ounces of pure water.

Body therapy: get twenty minutes of direct sunlight sometime during the day, but be careful between the hours of 10:00 a.m. and 2:00 p.m.

Breakfast

During breakfast, drink eight ounces of water or hot tea with honey (for recommended products, visit www.BiblicalHealthInstitute.com and click on the GPRx Resource Guide).

one bowl of organic "old-fashioned" whole oatmeal with honey, butter, cinnamon, and raisins with one tablespoon of extra virgin coconut oil and one- to- two tablespoons of protein powder (optional)

Supplements: take one to three liquid caps of an AM essential oil and a CO_2 blend of herbs and spices, and two whole food multivitamin caplets with zinc. (For recommended products, visit www.BiblicalHealth Institute.com and click on the GPRx Resource Guide.)

Lunch

Before eating, drink eight ounces of water.

one large bowl of Cold and Flu Bustin' Spicy Chicken Soup (see page 75 for recipe)

Supplements: take two whole food multivitamin caplets with zinc.

Dinner

Before eating, drink eight ounces of water.

During dinner, drink hot tea with honey

baked, poached, or grilled wild-caught salmon

stir-fried broccoli cooked in one tablespoon of extra virgin coconut oil

large green salad with mixed greens, avocado, carrots, cucumbers, celery, tomato, red cabbage, red onions, red peppers, and sprouts

salad dressing: extra virgin olive oil, apple cider vinegar or lemon juice, Celtic Sea Salt, herbs, and spices, or mix one tablespoon of extra virgin olive oil with one tablespoon of a healthy store-bought dressing

Supplements: take one to three liquid caps of a PM essential oil and a CO_2 blend of herbs and spices, two whole food multivitamin caplets, and one to three teaspoons or three to nine capsules of a high omega-3 cod-liver oil complex (for recommended products, visit www.Biblical HealthInstitute.com and click on the GPRx Resource Guide).

Snacks

apple slices with raw almond butter

one whole food nutrition bar with beta-glucans from soluble oat fiber (for recommended products, visit www.BiblicalHealthInstitute.com and click on the GPRx Resource Guide)

Drink eight to twelve ounces of water, or hot or iced fresh-brewed tea with honey.

Before Bed

Supplements: drink a mixture of two-to-three tablespoons of organic, unfiltered apple cider vinegar and one tablespoon of raw organic honey mixed in eight ounces of warm water. Take three-to-six caplets of a botanical herb and spice combination with garlic, ginger, elderberry, and echinacea with eight-to-twelve ounces of pure water.

Body therapy: take a warm bath for fifteen minutes with eight-to-twelve drops of biblical essential oils added (for recommended products, visit www.BiblicalHealthInstitute.com and click on the GPRx Resource Guide).

Advanced hygiene: repeat the advanced hygiene instructions from the morning of Day 1.

Prayer: thank God for this day, asking Him to give you a restoring night's rest and a fresh start tomorrow. Thank Him for His steadfast love that never ceases and His mercies new every morning. Read Romans 8:35, 37–39 out loud.

Sleep: go to bed by 10:30 p.m.

DAY 2

Upon Waking

Prayer: thank God because this is the day that the Lord has made. Rejoice and be glad in it. Thank Him for the breath in your lungs and the life in your body. Ask the Lord to heal your body. Read Psalm 91 out loud.

Advanced hygiene (you may practice advanced hygiene up to five times per day during a cold or flu): follow the advanced hygiene recommendations from the morning of Day 1.

Supplements: drink a mixture of two-to-three tablespoons of organic, unfiltered apple cider vinegar and one tablespoon of raw organic honey mixed in eight ounces of warm water. Take three-to-six caplets of a botanical herb and spice combination with garlic, ginger, elderberry, and echinacea with eight-to-twelve ounces of pure water.

Body therapy: take a hot and cold shower. After a normal shower, alternate sixty seconds of water as hot as you can stand it, followed by sixty seconds of water as cold as you can stand it. Repeat cycle seven-and-a-half times for a total of fifteen minutes, finishing with hot water.

Breakfast

Before eating, drink eight ounces of water.

During breakfast, drink eight ounces of water or hot tea with honey.

two or three eggs any style, cooked in one tablespoon of extra virgin coconut oil (for recommended products, visit www.BiblicalHealth Institute.com and click on the GPRx Resource Guide)

stir-fried onions, mushrooms, and peppers cooked in one tablespoon of extra virgin coconut oil

one slice of sprouted or yeast-free whole grain bread with almond butter and honey

Supplements: take one to three liquid caps of an AM essential oil and a CO_2 blend of herbs and spices (for recommended products, visit www.BiblicalHealthInstitute.com and click on the GPRx Resource Guide) and take two whole food multivitamin caplets with zinc.

Lunch

Before eating, drink eight ounces of water.

one large bowl of Cold and Flu Bustin' Spicy Chicken Soup (see page 75 for recipe)

Supplements: take two whole food multivitamin caplets with zinc.

Dinner

Before eating, drink eight ounces of water.

During dinner, drink hot tea with honey.

roasted organic chicken

cooked vegetables (carrots, onions, peas, etc.) cooked in one table-spoon of extra virgin coconut oil

large green salad with mixed greens, avocado, carrots, tomato, red cabbage, red onions, red peppers, and sprouts

salad dressing: extra virgin olive oil, apple cider vinegar or lemon juice, Celtic Sea Salt, herbs, and spices, or mix one tablespoon of extra virgin olive oil with one tablespoon of a healthy store-bought dressing

Supplements: take one to three liquid caps of a PM essential oil and a CO_2 blend of herbs and spices and two whole food multivitamin caplets and one to three teaspoons or three to nine capsules of a high omega-3 cod-liver oil complex.

Snacks

raw almonds and apple wedges

one whole food nutrition bar with beta-glucans from soluble oat fiber

Drink eight-to-twelve ounces of water, or hot or iced fresh-brewed tea with honey.

Before Bed

Supplements: drink a mixture of two-to-three tablespoons of organic, unfiltered apple cider vinegar and one tablespoon of raw organic honey mixed in eight ounces of warm water. Take three-to-six caplets of a botanical herb and spice combination with garlic, ginger, elderberry, and echinacea with eight-to-twelve ounces of pure water.

Advanced hygiene: repeat the advanced hygiene instructions from the morning of Day 1.

Prayer: thank God for this day, asking Him to give you a restoring night's rest and a fresh start tomorrow. Thank Him for His steadfast love that never ceases and His mercies new every morning. Read 1 Corinthians 13:4–8 out loud.

Body therapy: take a warm bath for fifteen minutes with eight-to-twelve drops of biblical essential oils added to the water.

Sleep: go to bed by 10:30 p.m.

DAY 3

Upon Waking

Prayer: thank God because this is the day that the Lord has made. Rejoice and be glad in it. Thank Him for the breath in your lungs and the life in your body. Ask the Lord to heal your body. Read Ephesians 6:13–18 out loud.

Advanced hygiene (you may practice advanced hygiene up to five times per day during a cold or flu): follow the advanced hygiene recommendations from the morning of Day 1.

Supplements: drink a mixture of two-to-three tablespoons of organic, unfiltered apple cider vinegar and one tablespoon of raw organic honey mixed in eight ounces of warm water. Take three-to-six caplets of a botanical herb and spice combination with garlic, ginger, elderberry, and echinacea with eight-to-twelve ounces of pure water.

Body therapy: take a hot and cold shower. After a normal shower, alternate sixty seconds of water as hot as you can stand it, followed by sixty seconds of water as cold as you can stand it. Repeat cycle seven-and-a-half times for a total of fifteen minutes, finishing with hot water.

Breakfast

During breakfast, drink eight ounces of water or hot tea with honey (for recommended products, visit www.BiblicalHealthInstitute.com and click on the GPRx Resource Guide).

one bowl of organic "old-fashioned" whole oatmeal with honey, butter, cinnamon, and raisins with one tablespoon of extra virgin coconut oil and one to two tablespoons of protein powder (optional)

Supplements: take one to three liquid caps of an AM essential oil and a CO_2 blend of herbs and spices (for recommended products, visit www.BiblicalHealthInstitute.com and click on the GPRx Resource Guide) and take two whole food multivitamin caplets with zinc.

Lunch

Before eating, drink eight ounces of water.

one large bowl of Cold and Flu Bustin' Spicy Chicken Soup (see page 75 for recipe)

Supplements: take two whole food multivitamin caplets with zinc.

Dinner

Before eating, drink eight ounces of water.

During dinner, drink hot tea with honey.

red meat steak (beef, buffalo, or venison)

sautéed broccoli cooked in one tablespoon of extra virgin coconut oil

baked sweet potato with butter

large green salad with mixed greens, avocado, carrots, cucumbers, celery, tomatoes, red cabbage, red peppers, red onions, and sprouts

salad dressing: extra virgin olive oil, apple cider vinegar or lemon juice, Celtic Sea Salt, herbs, and spices, or mix one tablespoon of extra virgin olive oil with one tablespoon of a healthy store-bought dressing

Supplements: take one to three liquid caps of a PM essential oil, a CO_2 blend of herbs and spices, two whole food multivitamin caplets, and one to three teaspoons or three to nine capsules of a high omega-3 cod-liver oil complex.

Snacks

one grapefruit or orange

one whole food nutrition bar with beta-glucans from soluble oat fiber

Drink eight to twelve ounces of water, or hot or iced fresh-brewed tea with honey.

Before Bed

Supplements: drink a mixture of two-to-three tablespoons of organic, unfiltered apple cider vinegar and one tablespoon of raw organic honey mixed in eight ounces of warm water. Take three-to-six caplets of a botanical herb and spice combination with garlic, ginger, elderberry, and echinacea with eight-to-twelve ounces of pure water.

Body therapy: take a warm bath for fifteen minutes with eight-to-twelve drops of biblical essential oils added to the water.

Advanced hygiene: follow the advanced hygiene instructions from the morning of Day 1.

Prayer: thank God for this day, asking Him to give you a restoring night's rest and a fresh start tomorrow. Thank Him for His steadfast love that never ceases and His mercies new every morning. Read Philippians 4:4–8, 11–13, 19 out loud.

Sleep: go to bed by 10:30 p.m.

Day 4

Upon Waking

Prayer: thank God because this is the day the Lord has made. Rejoice and be glad in it. Thank Him for the breath in your lungs and the life in your body. Read Matthew 6:9–13 out loud.

Advanced hygiene (you may practice advanced hygiene up to five times per day during a cold or flu): follow the advanced hygiene recommendations from Day 1.

Supplements: drink a mixture of two-to-three tablespoons of organic, unfiltered apple cider vinegar and one tablespoon of raw organic honey mixed in eight ounces of warm water. Take three-to-six caplets of a botanical herb and spice combination with garlic, ginger, elderberry, and echinacea with eight-to-twelve ounces of pure water.

Body therapy: take a hot and cold shower. After a normal shower, alternate sixty seconds of water as hot as you can stand it, followed by sixty seconds of water as cold as you can stand it. Repeat cycle seven and a half times for a total of fifteen minutes, finishing with hot water.

Breakfast

three soft-boiled or poached eggs

one grapefruit or orange

one cup of hot tea with honey

Supplements: take one to three liquid caps of an AM essential oil, a CO_2 blend of herbs and spices, and two whole food multivitamin caplets with zinc.

Lunch

Before eating, drink eight ounces of water.

one large bowl of Cold and Flu Bustin' Spicy Chicken Soup (see page 75 for recipe)

Supplements: take two whole food multivitamin caplets with zinc.

Dinner

Before eating, drink eight ounces of water.

During dinner, drink hot tea with honey.

grilled chicken breast

sautéed veggies cooked in one tablespoon of extra virgin coconut oil small portion of cooked non-gluten whole grain (quinoa, amaranth, millet, or buckwheat) cooked with one tablespoon of extra virgin coconut oil

large green salad with mixed greens, avocado, carrots, cucumbers, celery, tomatoes, red cabbage, red peppers, red onions, and sprouts

salad dressing: extra virgin olive oil, apple cider vinegar or lemon juice, Celtic Sea Salt, herbs, and spices, or mix one tablespoon of extra virgin olive oil with one tablespoon of a healthy store-bought dressing

Supplements: take one to three liquid caps of a PM essential oil and a CO_2 blend of herbs and spices, two whole food multivitamin caplets, and one to three teaspoons or three to nine capsules of a high omega-3 cod-liver oil complex.

Snacks

apple and carrots with raw almond butter

one whole food nutrition bar with beta-glucans from soluble oat fiber

Drink eight to twelve ounces of water, or hot or iced fresh-brewed tea with honey.

Before Bed

Drink eight-to-twelve ounces of water or hot tea with honey.

Supplements: drink a mixture of two-to-three tablespoons of organic, unfiltered apple cider vinegar and one tablespoon of raw organic honey mixed in eight ounces of warm water. Take three-to-six caplets of a botanical herb and spice combination with garlic, ginger, elderberry, and echinacea with eight-to-twelve ounces of pure water.

Advanced hygiene: follow the advanced hygiene recommendations from the morning of Day 1.

Prayer: thank God for this day, asking Him to give you a restoring night's rest and a fresh start tomorrow. Thank Him for His steadfast love that never ceases and His mercies that are new every morning. Read Romans 8:35, 37–39 out loud.

Body therapy: take a warm bath for fifteen minutes with eight-to-twelve drops of biblical essential oils added to the water.

Sleep: go to bed by 10:30 p.m.

DAY 5 (PARTIAL FAST DAY)

Upon Waking

Prayer: thank God because this is the day the Lord has made. Rejoice and be glad in it. Thank Him for the breath in your lungs and the life in your body. Read Isaiah 58:6–9 out loud.

Advanced hygiene (you may practice advanced hygiene up to five times per day during a cold or flu): follow the advanced hygiene recommendations from Day 1.

Supplements: drink a mixture of two-to-three tablespoons of organic, unfiltered apple cider vinegar and one tablespoon of raw organic honey mixed in eight ounces of warm water. Take three-to-six caplets of a botanical herb and spice combination with garlic, ginger, elderberry, and echinacea with eight-to-twelve ounces of pure water.

Body therapy: take a hot and cold shower. After a normal shower, alternate sixty seconds of water as hot as you can stand it, followed by sixty seconds of water as cold as you can stand it. Repeat cycle seven and a half times for a total of fifteen minutes, finishing with hot water.

Breakfast

none (partial fast day)

eight-to-twelve ounces of water

Supplements: take one to three liquid caps of an AM essential oil, a CO_2 blend of herbs and spices, and two whole food multivitamin caplets with zinc.

Lunch

none (partial fast day)

Supplements: take two whole food multivitamin caplets with zinc.

Dinner

Before eating, drink eight ounces of water.

During dinner, drink hot tea with honey.

one large bowl of Cold and Flu Bustin' Spicy Chicken Soup (see page 75 for recipe)

cultured vegetables (for recommended products, visit www.Biblical HealthInstitute.com and click on the GPRx Resource Guide)

large green salad with mixed greens, avocado, carrots, cucumbers, celery, tomatoes, red cabbage, red peppers, red onions, and sprouts

salad dressing: extra virgin olive oil, apple cider vinegar or lemon juice, Celtic Sea Salt, herbs, and spices, or mix one tablespoon of extra virgin olive oil with one tablespoon of a healthy store-bought dressing

Supplements: take Take one- to- three liquid caps of a PM essential oil, a CO_2 blend of herbs and spices, two whole food multivitamin caplets, and one to three teaspoons or three to nine capsules of a high omega-3 cod-liver oil complex.

Snacks

none (partial fast day)

drink eight ounces of water

Before Bed

Drink eight-to-twelve ounces of water or hot tea with honey.

Supplements: drink a mixture of two-to-three tablespoons of organic, unfiltered apple cider vinegar and one tablespoon of raw organic honey mixed in eight ounces of warm water. Take three-to-six caplets of a botanical herb and spice combination with garlic, ginger, elderberry, and echinacea with eight-to-twelve ounces of pure water.

Advanced hygiene: follow the advanced hygiene recommendations from the morning of Day 1.

Body therapy: take a warm bath for fifteen minutes with eight-to-twelve drops of biblical essential oils added to the water.

Prayer: thank God for this day, asking Him to give you a restoring night's rest and a fresh start tomorrow. Thank Him for His steadfast love that never ceases and His mercies that are new every morning. Read Isaiah 58:6–9 out loud.

Sleep: go to bed by 10:30 p.m.

Day 6

Upon Waking

Prayer: thank God because this is the day the Lord has made. Rejoice and be glad in it. Thank Him for the breath in your lungs and the life in your body. Read Psalm 23 out loud.

Advanced hygiene (you may practice advanced hygiene up to five times per day during a cold or flu): follow the advanced hygiene recommendations from Day 1.

Supplements: drink a mixture of two-to-three tablespoons of organic, unfiltered apple cider vinegar and one tablespoon of raw organic honey mixed in eight ounces of warm water. Take three-to-six caplets of a botanical herb and spice combination with garlic, ginger, elderberry, and echinacea with eight-to-twelve ounces of pure water.

Body therapy: take a hot and cold shower. After a normal shower, alternate sixty seconds of water as hot as you can stand it, followed by sixty seconds of water as cold as you can stand it. Repeat cycle seven-and-a-half times for a total of fifteen minutes, finishing with hot water.

Breakfast

two or three eggs cooked any style in one tablespoon of extra virgin coconut oil

one grapefruit or orange

handful of almonds

Supplements: take one to three liquid caps of an AM essential oil, a CO_2 blend of herbs and spices, and two whole food multivitamin caplets with zinc.

Lunch

Before eating, drink eight ounces of water.

one large bowl of Cold and Flu Bustin' Spicy Chicken Soup (see page 75 for recipe)

Supplements: take two whole food multivitamin caplets with zinc.

Dinner

Before eating, drink eight ounces of water.

During dinner, drink hot tea with honey.

roasted organic chicken

sautéed vegetables (carrots, onions, peas, etc.) cooked in one tablespoon of extra virgin coconut oil

large green salad with mixed greens, carrots, cucumbers, celery, tomatoes, red cabbage, red peppers, red onions, and sprouts

salad dressing: extra virgin olive oil, apple cider vinegar or lemon juice, Celtic Sea Salt, herbs, and spices, or mix one tablespoon of extra virgin olive oil with one tablespoon of a healthy store-bought dressing

Supplements: take Take one- to- three liquid caps of a PM essential oil, a CO_2 blend of herbs and spices, two whole food multivitamin caplets, and one to three teaspoons or three to nine capsules of a high omega-3 cod-liver oil complex.

Snacks

handful of raw almonds with apple wedges

one whole food nutrition bar with beta-glucans from soluble oat fiber

Drink eight to twelve ounces of water, or hot or iced fresh-brewed tea with honey.

Before Bed

Drink eight-to-twelve ounces of water or hot tea with honey.

Supplements: drink a mixture of two-to-three tablespoons of organic, unfiltered apple cider vinegar and one tablespoon of raw organic honey mixed in eight ounces of warm water. Take three-to-six caplets of a botanical herb and spice combination with garlic, ginger, elderberry, and echinacea with eight-to-twelve ounces of pure water.

Advanced hygiene: follow the advanced hygiene recommendations from the morning of Day 1.

Prayer: thank God for this day, asking Him to give you a restoring night's rest and a fresh start tomorrow. Thank Him for His steadfast love that never ceases and His mercies that are new every morning. Read Psalm 23 out loud.

Body therapy: take a warm bath for fifteen minutes with eight-to-twelve drops of biblical essential oils added to the water.

Sleep: go to bed by 10:30 p.m.

DAY 7

Upon Waking

Prayer: thank God because this is the day that the Lord has made. Rejoice and be glad in it. Thank Him for the breath in your lungs and the life in your body. Read Psalm 91 out loud.

Advanced hygiene (you may practice advanced hygiene up to five times per day during a cold or flu): follow the advanced hygiene recommendations from Day 1.

Supplements: drink a mixture of two-to-three tablespoons of organic, unfiltered apple cider vinegar and one tablespoon of raw organic honey mixed in eight ounces of warm water. Take three-to-six caplets of a botanical herb and spice combination with garlic, ginger, elderberry, and echinacea with eight-to-twelve ounces of pure water.

Body therapy: take a hot and cold shower. After a normal shower, alternate sixty seconds of water as hot as you can stand it, followed by sixty seconds of water as cold as you can stand it. Repeat cycle seven-and-a-half times for a total of fifteen minutes, finishing with hot water.

Breakfast

During breakfast, drink eight ounces of water or hot tea with honey.

one bowl of organic "old-fashioned" whole oatmeal with honey, butter, cinnamon, and raisins, and one tablespoon of extra virgin coconut oil and one-to-two tablespoons of protein powder (optional)

Supplements: take one to three liquid caps of an AM essential oil, a CO_2 blend of herbs and spices, and two whole food multivitamin caplets with zinc.

Lunch

Before eating, drink eight ounces of water.

one large bowl of Cold and Flu Bustin' Spicy Chicken Soup see page 75 for recipe)

Supplements: take Take two whole food multivitamin caplets with zinc.

Dinner

Before eating, drink eight ounces of water.

During dinner, drink hot tea with honey.

baked or grilled fish of your choice

sautéed broccoli cooked in one tablespoon of extra virgin coconut oil

baked sweet potato with butter

large green salad with mixed greens, carrots, cucumbers, celery, tomatoes, red cabbage, red peppers, red onions, and sprouts salad dressing: extra virgin olive oil, apple cider vinegar or lemon juice, Celtic Sea Salt, herbs, and spices, or mix one tablespoon of extra virgin olive oil with one tablespoon of a healthy store-bought dressing

Supplements: take one to three liquid caps of a PM essential oil, a CO_2 blend of herbs and spices, and whole food multivitamin caplets, and one to three teaspoons or three to nine capsules of a high omega-3 cod-liver oil complex.

Snacks

apple slices with raw sesame butter (tahini)

one whole food nutrition bar with beta-glucans from soluble oat fiber

Drink eight to twelve ounces of water, or hot or iced fresh-brewed tea with honey.

Before Bed

Drink eight-to-twelve ounces of water or hot tea with honey.

Supplements: drink a mixture of two-to-three tablespoons of organic, unfiltered apple cider vinegar and one tablespoon of raw organic honey mixed in eight ounces of warm water. Take three-to-six caplets of a botanical herb and spice combination with garlic, ginger, elderberry, and echinacea with eight-to-twelve ounces of pure water.

Advanced hygiene: follow the advanced hygiene recommendations from the morning of Day 1.

Body therapy: take a warm bath for fifteen minutes with eight-to-twelve drops of biblical essential oils added to the water.

Prayer: thank God for this day, asking Him to give you a restoring night's rest and a fresh start tomorrow. Thank Him for His steadfast love that never ceases and His mercies that are new every morning. Read 1 Corinthians 13:4–8 out loud.

Sleep: go to bed by 10:30 p.m.

DAY 8 AND BEYOND

After you've recovered from your cold or flu and you want to continue to live a healthy life, visit www.GreatPhysiciansRx.com and join the 7 Weeks of Wellness online community, where you will learn detailed step-by-step suggestions and meal and lifestyle plans for healthy living. These online programs will also provide you with the tools to track your progress.

If you've experienced positive results from the Great Physician's Rx for Colds and Flu program, I encourage you to reach out to someone you know and recommend this book and program to them. You can learn how to lead a small group at your church or home by visiting www.GreatPhysiciansRx.com.

Remember: You don't have to be a doctor or a health expert to help transform the life of someone you care about—you just have to be willing.

Allow me to offer you this prayer of blessing paraphrased from Numbers 6:24–26:

May the Lord bless you and keep you.
May the Lord make His face to shine upon you and be
*   gracious unto you.*
May the Lord lift up His countenance upon you and bring you
*   peace.*
In the name of Yeshua Ha Mashiach, Jesus our Messiah.
Amen.

Need Recipes?

For a detailed list of more than two hundred healthy and delicious recipes contained in the Great Physician's Rx eating plan, please visit www.GreatPhysiciansRx.com.

Notes

Introduction

1. "The Influenza Pandemic of 1918," by Molly Billings and posted on the Stanford University Web site at www.stanford.edu/group/virus/uda.

2. *60 Minutes* broadcast of "Chasing the Flu," December 4, 2005.

3. Emily Flynn Vencat, "Public Health: No Cause for Panic," *Newsweek*, 24 October 2005.

4. "How to Avoid—Gesundheit!—the Cold and Flu," by Amy Cox of cnn.com and available at www.cnn.com/2004/HEALTH/12/13/cold.flu.overview.

5. "Children's Illnesses: Top Four Causes of Missed School," an article on the MayoClinic.com Web site and available at www.mayoclinic.com/health/childrens-conditions/CC00059.

6. "The Common Cold Coughs Ups a $40 Billion Annual Price Tag," a press release from the University of Michigan Health System, February 24, 2003, and available at http://www.med.umich.edu/opm/newspage/2003/cold.htm

7. "Cold Comfort: Cure Won't Be Soon," by Tal Mekel at cnn.com, December 15, 2004, and available at www.cnn.com/2004/HEALTH/12/13/cold.flu.cure.

8. Influenza statistics found on the Mayo Clinic Web site at http://www.mayoclinic.com/health/influenza/DS00081.

9. E. Cheraskin, MD, *Vitamin C: Who Needs It?* (Birmingham, AL: Arlington Press, 1993).

10. "Cold Comfort: Cure Won't Be Soon," by Tal Mekel at cnn.com, December 15, 2004, and available at http://www.cnn.com/2004/HEALTH/12/13/cold.flu.cure.

11. B. Braunig, et al., "*Echinacea purpurea radix* for Strengthening the Immune Response in Flu-Like Infections," *Z Phytother* 13 (1992): 7–13.

12. Phyllis A. Balch, CNC, *Prescription for Nutritional Healing* (Wayne, NJ: Avery Publishing, 2003), 298.

Key #1

1. "Is It 'Feed a Cold, Starve a Fever,' or Vice Versa?" *The Straight Dope* question-and-answer column, written by Cecil Adams and published by the *Chicago Reader* on May 3, 1996.

2. G.R., Van den Brink, et al., "Feed a Cold, Starve a Fever?" Clinical and Diagnostic Laboratory Immunology, 9 182–83 (2003), *Nature* 2002.

3. Larry Trivieri Jr., ed., *Alternative Medicine: The Definitive Guide* (Berkeley, CA: Celestial Arts, 2002), 675.

4. Dr. Appleton listed three sources for this dramatic statement: A. Sanchez, et al., "Role of Sugars in Human Neutrophilic Phagocytosis," *American Journal of Clinical Nutrition* 261 (November 1973): 1180–84; J. Bernstein, et al., "Depression of Lymphocyte Transformation Following Oral Glucose Ingestion," *American Journal of Clinical Nutrition* 30 (1997): 613; and W. Ringsdorf, E. Cheraskin, and R. Ramsay, "Sucrose, Neutrophilic Phagocytosis and Resistance to Disease," *Dental Survey* 52 (1976): 46–48.

5. Elena Gaona, "Ladling Up Comfort," *San Diego Union-Tribune*, 22 December 2005.

6. "Chicken Soup, Rx for the Cold," printed on the healthatoz.com Web site and available at www.healthatoz.com/healthatoz/Atoz/dc/caz/resp/cold/chixsoup.jsp.

7. The citation for Dr. Rennard's study: B.O. Rennard, et al., "Chicken Soup Inhibits Neutrophil Chemotaxis in Vitro," *Chest* 2000 November; 118(4): 1150–57.

8. James J. Gormley, "Pow! Why Everyone's Favorite Bulb Packs a Mean Punch—Immune-Boosting—Frontiers of Science," *Better Nutrition*, November 2001, and available online at www.findarticles.com/p/articles/mi_m0FKA/is_11_63/ai_83076750.

9. Paul Schulick, *Ginger: Common Spice & Wonder Drug*, Third Edition (Prescott, AZ: Hohm Press, 1996), 37.

Key #2

1. Linus Pauling, *Vitamin C and the Common Cold* (New York: W.H. Freeman & Co., 1970).

2. *Alternative Medicine: The Definitive Guide* (Celestial Arts, 2002) pointed to research published in E. Cheraskin, MD's book, *Vitamin C: Who Needs It?* (Arlington Press, 1993).

3. Michael Murray, ND, and Joseph Pizzorno, ND, *Encyclopedia of Natural Medicine*, (New York: Three Rivers Press, 1998), 373.

4. http://lpi.oregonstate.edu/infocenter/vitamins/vitaminC/

5. "Cold and Flu Health" by Christina Whitford in *Health Journal*, and available online at www.bodyandfitness.com/Information/Health/cold.htm#Elderberry's.

6. "Randomized Study of the Efficacy and Safety of Oral Elderberry Extract in the Treatment of Influenza A and B Virus Infections," *Journal of International Medicine*, J Int Med Res 2004;32(2):132–140.

Key #3

1. Kenneth Seaton, PhD, "A New Way to Prevent Colds and Flu," *Health Freedom News*, March 1992, 14.

2. From a 2003 study sponsored by the American Society for Microbiology as part of its "Take Action: Clean Hands Campaign," http://www.asm.org/Media/index.asp?bid=21773.

3. Jennifer Barrett Ozols, "Surviving the Sick Office," *Newsweek*, 22 March 2005.

Key #4

1. C. E. Matthews, I. S. Ockene, P. S. Freedson, M. C. Rosal, P. A. Merriam, and J. R. Hebert. "Moderate to vigorous physical activity and risk of upper-respiratory tract infection." *Med. Sci. Sports Exerc.*, Vol. 34, No. 8, pp. 1242–8, 2002.

2. Phyllis A. Balch, *Prescription for Nutritional Healing* (Wayne, NJ: Avery Publishing, 2003), 298.

Key #5

1. Jessica Nutik Zitter, MD, MPH; Peter D. Mazonson, MD, MBA; Dave P. Miller, MS; Stephen B. Hulley, MD, MPH; John R. Balmes, MD, "Aircraft Cabin Air Recirculation and Symptoms of a Common Cold," *JAMA.* 2002; 288:483–6.

2. Ibid.

Key #6

1. "Gesundheit!" an article written by *Psychology Today* staff members, *Psychology Today*, 1 November 2001.

2. "Beat the Winter Bugs: How to Hold Your Own Against Colds and Flu," U.S. Food and Drug Administration's *FDA Consumer* magazine, November-December 2001 issue.

3. Colin Allen, "Attitude Fights Colds," *Psychology Today*, 24 July 2003.

Key #7

1. "Nation's Leading Alarmists Excited About Bird Flu," an article on The Onion Web site, February 2, 2005, Issue 41-05, and available at www.theonion.com/content/node/30868.

About the Authors

Jordan Rubin has dedicated his life to transforming the health of others one life at a time. He is the founder and chairman of Garden of Life, Inc., a health and wellness company based in West Palm Beach, Florida, that produces whole food nutritional supplements and personal care products. He is also president and CEO of GPRx, Inc., a biblically based health and wellness company providing educational resources, small group curriculum, functional foods, nutritional supplements, and wellness services.

He and his wife, Nicki, married in 1999 and are the parents of a toddler-aged son, Joshua. They make their home in Palm Beach Gardens, Florida.

Joseph D. Brasco, M.D., has extensive knowledge and experience in gastroenterology and internal medicine. He attended medical school at Medical College of Wisconsin in Milwaukee, Wisconsin, and is board certified with the American Board of Internal Medicine. Besides writing for various medical journals, he is also the coauthor of *Restoring Your Digestive Health* with Jordan Rubin.

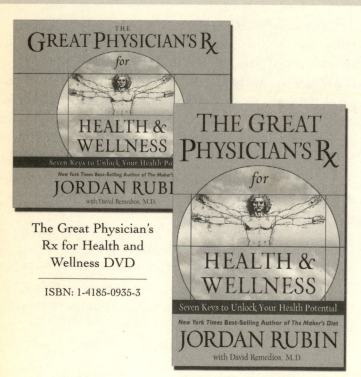

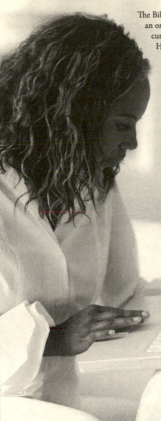

BHI

BIBLICAL HEALTH
INSTITUTE

The Biblical Health Institute (www.BiblicalHealthInstitute.com) is an online learning community housing educational resources and curricula reinforcing and expanding on Jordan Rubin's Biblical Health message.

Biblical Health Institute provides:

1. "101" level **FREE**, introductory courses corresponding to Jordan's book The Great Physician's Rx for Health and Wellness and its seven keys; Current "101" courses include:

   * "Eating to Live 101"

   * "Whole Food Nutrition Supplements 101"

   * "Advanced Hygiene 101"

   * "Exercise and Body Therapies 101"

   * "Reducing Toxins 101"

   * "Emotional Health 101"

   * "Prayer and Purpose 101"

2. **FREE** resources (healthy recipes, what to E.A.T., resource guide)

3. **FREE** media--videos and video clips of Jordan, music therapy samples, etc.--and much more!

Additionally, Biblical Health Institute also offers in-depth courses for those who want to go deeper.

Course offerings include:

   * 40-hour certificate program to become a Biblical Health Coach

   * A la carte course offerings designed for personal study and growth (launching late April 2006)

   * Home school courses developed by Christian educators, supporting home-schooled students and their parents (designed for middle school and high school ages—launching in August 2006).

**For more information and updates on these and other resources go to
www.BiblicalHealthInstitute.com**

EXPERIENCE
THE GREAT PHYSICIAN'S Rx
ONLINE

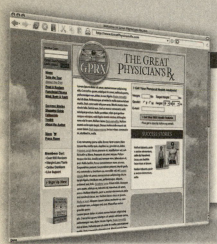

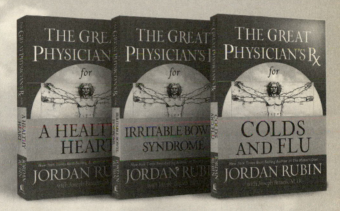

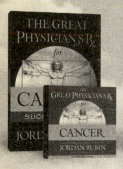 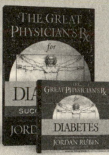 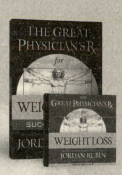

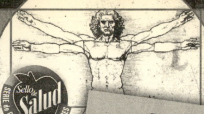
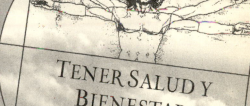